EATING WISELY AND WELL

Educated at the All India Institute of Medical Sciences and Massachusetts Institute of Technology, **Dr Ramesh Bijlani**, MD; SM; DSc (Honoris causa); FAMS, spent twenty-five years researching on nutrition in relation to cardiovascular disease and diabetes. At the same time, since 1992, he has delved into the depths of yoga, specially the integral yoga of Sri Aurobindo and the Mother. His intimate contact with ancient Indian wisdom has made him aware of the lacunae in the modern science of nutrition, and how these may be filled up by turning to Ayurveda and yoga. He is also the author of *Back to Health through Yoga*.

Eating Wisely and Well is the essence of good nutrition practice and philosophy. Dr Bijlani's rich experience and sensitivity to value-based life helps enunciate the basic principles of nutrition.

Anupa Siddhu, PhD
Director, Lady Irwin College

Eating Wisely and Well is not only relishing and refreshing, but also reassuring and uplifting. Springing forth from the pen of a reputed nutrition scientist, who is well versed in both modern scientific medical investigations and traditional systems of Yoga and Ayurveda, this book spans a wide breadth of knowledge on many important aspects of human nutrition. [...] a must read for people who want to know 'what to eat' and 'how to eat'.

A. J. Vinaya Simha, MD
Professor of Endocrinology,
Texas Tech University Health Center

Like Dr Bijlani's earlier books, *Eating Wisely and Well* is superbly written, scientifically accurate, and holistic in nature. The lucid style will appeal to a wide array of readers. Practical tips in every chapter will help and guide healthy eating behaviours.

Sakti Srivastava, MBBS, MS
Associate Professor of Surgery,
Stanford University School of Medicine

This book will not only appeal to the layperson, but will also be a useful adjunct for the students and practitioners of medicine.

C. S. Pandav, MD
Professor and Head,
Centre for Community Medicine, AIIMS

EATING WISELY AND WELL

Ramesh Bijlani

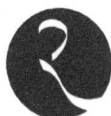

RUPA

First published in 2012 by
Rupa Publications India Pvt. Ltd.
7/16, Ansari Road, Daryaganj,
New Delhi 110 002

Sales Centres:

Allahabad Bengaluru Chennai
Hyderabad Jaipur Kathmandu
Kolkata Mumbai

10 9 8 7 6 5 4 3 2 1

Ramesh Bijlani asserts the moral right to be
identified as the author of this work.

Printed at Repro Knowledgecast Limited, Thane

To
LOVLEEN

getting married to whom
was the best thing that
happened to me in life

I, having become the flame of life (Vaishvaanara), established into the body of living creatures and united with Praana and Apaana (the incoming and outgoing breath), digest the four kinds of food.

BHAGAVAD GITA, 15:14

It is the attachment to food, the greed and eagerness for it, making it an unduly important thing in the life, that is contrary to the spirit of yoga. To be aware that something is pleasant to the palate is not wrong; only one must have no desire nor hankering for it, no exultation in getting it, no displeasure or regret at not getting it. [...] To be always thinking about food and troubling the mind is quite the wrong way of getting rid of the food-desire. Put the food element in the right place in the life, in a small corner, and don't concentrate on it but on other things.

SRI AUROBINDO

The all-absorbing interest which nearly all human beings, even the most intellectual, have in food, its preparation and its consumption, should be replaced by an almost chemical knowledge of the needs of the body and a very scientific austerity in satisfying them.

THE MOTHER
(of Sri Aurobindo Ashram)

Contents

Preface

Getting into the Spirit of the Book

One should not eat in order to please the palate, but just to keep the body going. When each organ of sense subserves the body, and through the body the soul, its special relish disappears and then alone does it begin to function in the way nature intended it to.

MAHATMA GANDHI

One way of looking at life is as a series of choices, and we can exercise those choices at different levels. For example, when it comes to food, we may choose primarily from the emotional level and eat what we find good to taste. Alternatively, we may rise to the rational level and eat what is in the best interests of good health. For this, we need to know what benefits different foods provide us and what our requirements are. The science of nutrition, which embodies this knowledge, is still incomplete, but is growing and constantly getting better. The principal goal of this book is to give the reader the current scientific knowledge about nutrition in a way that is easy to understand and also easy to apply in daily life. The good news is that eating a healthy diet is simple, especially for Indians, because a good traditional Indian diet meets our requirements in terms of current scientific knowledge exceedingly well.

When it comes to making choices, it is also possible to rise above the rational, access the deepest part of our being and make a choice based on love and compassion. Doing so in relation to food leads us to choices which are not only healthy but also ethical and eco-friendly. One who makes such choices becomes not just physically healthy but also enjoys inner peace and well-being. This is an aspect of nutrition that goes beyond what is strictly scientific, but is a part of wisdom traditions.

The three levels of decision-making: emotional, rational and supra-rational, are neither totally unrelated, nor necessarily in conflict with one another. A healthy, ethical and eco-friendly diet can also be very palatable. This book aims at facilitating food choices that are not only scientifically sound but also satisfactory from every other angle. Moderation, not monasticism, is the thrust of this book, and not just because monasticism does not suit most of us. Intolerable dos and don'ts about foods are impressive, but neither necessary nor desirable. The mental stress created by denial and deprivation may do more harm to physical health than the good that eating by the rule book might do. Prolonged fasts and punishing food regimens in the name of spiritual discipline might generate deadly spiritual pride rather than spiritual progress.

The first book that I wrote was also a popular book on nutrition. It was published in 1974 under the title *Eating Scientifically*, and has long been out of print. In the thirty-eight years since that book was published, the science of nutrition has grown, food choices have changed and hopefully, with the passing years, I have acquired not only experience but also some more knowledge and wisdom. I am pleased to share with the readers my current perception of a subject which is a major preoccupation of man. Readers may feel free to send me comments and suggestions for further improving this book, by writing to me at rambij@gmail.com.

1
Asking the Right Questions

A question that sometimes drives me hazy: am I or are the others crazy?

ALBERT EINSTEIN

Of all my popular lectures, those on nutrition are followed by the longest question–answer sessions. The positive side of these marathon sessions is that people are immensely interested in knowing more about what they eat, and realize the value of food for staying healthy as well as for treating disease. But the nature of the questions often reveals that their curiosity is misdirected due to the vast amount of information and misinformation that they already have about the details, while they are quite ignorant about basic broad principles.

The largest category of questions is about individual foods. For example, one person may ask if olive oil is the best oil while another might want to know whether green tea is good for the heart. Strictly speaking, these questions need only a 'Yes' or a 'No', but in fact, it is impossible to give such an answer for a variety of reasons. First, no single food is so good as to compensate for all the defects of a faulty diet. Second, too much of a good food (e.g. milk) may be harmful, and a little bit of supposedly harmful foods (e.g. sugar or salt) may be quite harmless. If a food was so bad that even occasional use of a little bit of it could cause serious harm, it would have by now been classified as a poison. Third, no food is indispensable. If some food can make a valuable contribution to diet but happens to be exotic or expensive, it can generally be replaced by simpler, cheaper and easily available substitutes. Finally, the golden rule of nutrition is that a good diet should have a variety of foods. Of course, the variety should be judiciously chosen. But too much should not be expected of individual foods. Miracle foods just do not exist.

Several questions originate from our tendency to cling to long-cherished myths, especially myths that were once considered facts. These questions are asked with the fond hope that the expert will confirm the myth; the questioner almost tries to put words into the expert's mouth. For example, people refuse to accept that cereals are a major source of protein in an Indian vegetarian diet, that a cereal–pulse mixture can meet all of our protein requirements, and that even children do not need any protein-rich foods, such as eggs or meat. In order to learn more, we should be ready to unlearn outdated clichés, myths and superstitions.

Yet another category of questions arises from reports in the media based on single studies. Even if a study has been conducted at a reputed centre and has been published in a prestigious journal, it rarely qualifies as popular science. There are often some vested interests behind the undue publicity that some single studies get. A careful and critical reader should remember that sound scientific advice on nutrition today is based on the synthesis of thousands of studies that have been conducted over the last three centuries or so. Sometimes, even all this accumulated information is not enough, and we also need to consider the time-honoured wisdom that has been gleaned over thousands of years, and has now become a part of our venerable cultures. While a single study may state a truth, even under the best of circumstances, its truth is only a very, very tiny part of the whole truth. Under circumstances that are not so good, the conclusions of the study may be based on erroneous interpretation of observations, and the interpretation may be refuted by another subsequent study.

I have never really understood why the general public has a tendency to complicate the simple task of eating well. Sometimes, they complicate it by insisting on trivial details, refusing to believe that such details are inconsequential. At other times, they complicate the task by imposing on themselves unnecessary restrictions. Occasionally, they punish themselves due to their unwillingness to digest a little necessary complexity. A case in point is diabetes. So many diabetics feel they have done all that is necessary if they have given up consuming sugar. They forget that management of diabetes is not so simple. First, if they understand the principles of nutrition well, they can enjoy sugar in moderation. Second, they can eat a fairly 'normal' diet, which would be a healthy diet even for the rest of the family. Third, in addition to the diet, exercise and mental relaxation are also important lifestyle measures for the treatment of diabetes. Finally, neither do lifestyle measures always eliminate the need for medication, nor does medication ever eliminate the need for a healthy lifestyle.

There is absolutely no doubt that food is a major lifestyle determinant of health and disease. The effect of food on health depends on at least three factors. The first of these is *what* we eat. This is the factor that gets maximum attention. The second factor is *how much* we eat, and how much of each food we eat. This factor gets less attention than it deserves. Finally, the *attitude* with which we eat also influences the effect of food on us. This factor hardly gets any attention, but is no less powerful just because it is intangible. If we direct our attention towards these three factors, we can hope to get the right answers for getting the maximum from our food in terms of our total well-being.

SUMMARY

1. We often complicate the task of eating well by asking the wrong questions.
2. Instead of concentrating on single foods and classifying them into good and bad foods, it is better to focus on the diet as a whole. No single food is so good as to compensate

for all the defects of a faulty diet. Further, too much of a good food may be harmful, and a little bit of even a notorious food may be quite harmless. Finally, miracle foods just do not exist.

3. In order to learn more, we should be ready to unlearn some long-cherished beliefs if they are not true.

4. Sound advice on nutrition cannot be based on single research studies.

5. We need not insist on trivial, inconsequential details, or impose on ourselves unnecessary dietary restrictions. Sometimes, we should also be ready to digest a little necessary complexity.

6. How our diet affects us depends on what we eat, how much we eat and the attitude with which we eat.

2
Cinderella

Blessed are the meek, for they shall inherit the earth.

THE BIBLE (Matthew 5:5)

The subject of nutrition is best approached in terms of nutrients. Nutrients are the classes of chemical compounds that are present in foods. The reason why this approach is better than talking about foods directly may be easily understood through a simple analogy. Starting with a few types of yarn, such as cotton, silk, wool and polyester, we manufacture a wide variety of textiles. Further, these textiles may be cut and stitched in different ways to give us a still wider variety of garments. Similarly, various permutations and combinations of just a few nutrients make up a wide variety of foods. Further, by cooking and processing these foods in different ways, we get a still wider variety of recipes. Therefore, if we start with nutrients, the task of understanding the science of nutrition becomes much simpler. Although our foods come in a bewildering variety, the process of digestion breaks them up into their constituent nutrients. Since foods are eventually absorbed by the body as nutrients, and it is nutrients that the body needs, understanding foods in terms of their nutrient composition simplifies the task of eating a satisfactory diet. For example, a rice-eater will not complain if he is given only wheat, and someone accustomed to yellow gram will not complain if he gets red gram instead, provided the primary concern is satisfactory nutrient intake, rather than taste or habit*. Wheat offers the same nutrients as rice, and the nutrient composition of yellow gram does not differ much from that of red gram. An Indian diet looks so different from a European or Chinese diet, but they all supply the same set of nutrients. With some knowledge of the nutrient composition of foods, any of these diets can be tailored to provide a person with all the necessary nutrients in the right quantity. Not knowing chemistry is not a handicap to understanding the science of nutrition in terms of nutrients. In order to drive a car, or even to be a good car mechanic, it is not necessary to be an automobile engineer. This chapter will discuss just one nutrient—carbohydrates.

The humble carbohydrates are the Cinderella of nutrition. About 70 per cent of the energy content of an Indian diet comes from carbohydrates. Yet, carbohydrates are often looked down upon as a necessary evil. Indians

---

*An exception would be a person who is allergic to wheat. He is fully justified in refusing to eat wheat.

have a tendency to blame poverty and poor traditions for the high carbohydrate content of their diets. Affluent Indians often declare with an air of superiority, 'I eat no carbs', little realizing that if it is really so, they are eating very poorly indeed. The science of nutrition can today safely assert that if 70 per cent of one's energy comes from carbohydrates, it is an indicator of a healthy diet.

Dietary carbohydrates are either starches (complex carbohydrates) or sugars (simple carbohydrates). The principal sources of starch are cereals, pulses, potatoes and bananas. Only two sugars are nutritionally significant: cane sugar (sucrose) and milk sugar (lactose).

It is a common misconception that cereals, such as wheat, rice, barley, maize, etc. have starch, whereas pulses (dals) or legumes, such as green gram, red gram, bengal gram, kidney beans, etc. have protein. In fact, a typical cereal contains about 70 per cent, by weight, of carbohydrates, whereas a typical pulse has about 60 per cent, by weight, of carbohydrates. Cereals and pulses constitute the major source of carbohydrates in a good Indian diet.

Are all carbohydrates alike?

All carbohydrates provide 4 Calories per gram. Thus, one teaspoon of sugar, which weighs 5 grams, gives 20 Calories. In spite of this basic similarity, there are several reasons why the type and source of carbohydrates does matter. From the nutritional angle, the all-important comparison is between starch and sugar.

Starch comes with a bonus

Most of our dietary starch comes from cereals and pulses. Cereals and pulses are a package deal. They provide not only carbohydrates but also protein, a small quantity (but an important type) of fat, some vitamins, some minerals and so on. It is impossible to get carbohydrates from cereals or pulses without obtaining the other nutrients as well. Thus, eating cereals and pulses automatically ensures a supply of several other nutrients, which we also need. In contrast, sugar is 100 per cent carbohydrate. For once, such purity is not desirable; it is much better to take carbohydrates 'contaminated' with protein, fat, vitamins and minerals.

Whither blood sugar?

A healthy person who has not eaten for four hours or more has a blood sugar level of about 100 mg/dL. If such a person eats a meal, the carbohydrate in his food yields glucose upon digestion. The glucose crosses the intestinal wall and enters the blood stream. The rate at which glucose is released into the blood stream is influenced by the type of carbohydrate in the meal. Starch needs much more elaborate digestion than sugar. Therefore, glucose is delivered to the blood slowly from starch, whereas it is delivered rather rapidly from sugar. The result is that the blood sugar level rises faster, and to a higher peak level, after eating sugar, than after eating the same amount of carbohydrate in the form of starch (Fig. 2.1). This makes starch a much better choice than sugar from the point of view of prevention or management of diabetes.*

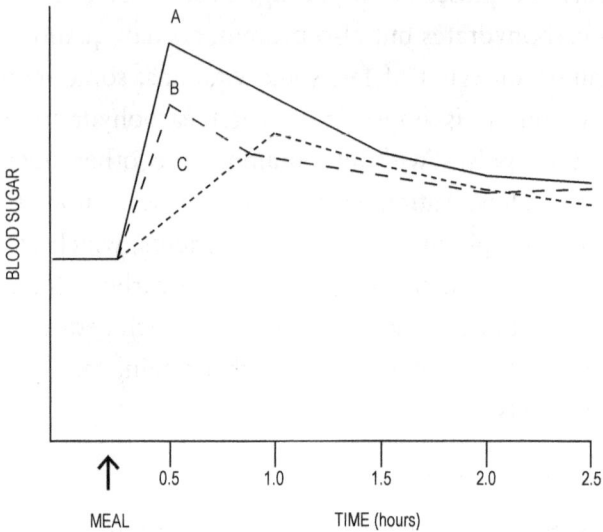

Fig. 2.1. The rise in blood sugar after three meals, which have exactly the same amount of carbohydrate. (A) Sugar; (B) Starch; (C) Unrefined starchy food grain.

---

*Besides giving preference to starch as compared to sugar, there are several other dietary choices that help in reducing the fasting as well as postprandial (after meals) blood sugar levels. Some of these are: consuming more dietary fibre, eating more of pulses, and having small frequent meals instead of a single large meal.

The calorie count

Although starch and sugar both give 4 Calories for each gram consumed, the energy we get depends on the quantity we consume. Starchy foods take time and effort to chew, and therefore, we feel satisfied after eating an amount that is pretty well matched with our requirements. In contrast, sugar-containing foods (e.g. sweets, cake and ice cream) are palatable and easy to eat. They are often eaten after a full meal, and are thus unwanted extras. The result is that sugar encourages us to overeat. Overeating happens even when the sugary food itself is the meal, and not an extra. Imagine eating a meal which has brown bread or brown rice, and a meal which has just cake. One is sure to consume far more calories in the meal consisting entirely of cake.

The cavity count

Just as we love sugar, the germs that live in our mouth also love it. When we have a sugar-heavy meal, we inevitably share it with the germs, especially if the food is sticky (e.g. chocolate) and we leave it stuck between the teeth for long. Sharing food with our microscopic guests may be generous, but these guests do not behave well. In the process of utilizing the sugar, they spill acid on our teeth. Acid eats away the teeth's outermost protective covering (enamel). The process gradually leads to the formation of tiny pits, called cavities. A pit that finally becomes deep enough to expose the nerve endings at the bottom of the teeth becomes painful. For preventing cavities, two precautions are very important. First, avoid foods containing sugar, especially those which are likely to get stuck between the teeth. Second, wash your mouth thoroughly immediately after a meal; rather, after eating anything at all, even if it is a snack or just a biscuit. Immediately after eating means absolutely immediately— even a delay of a few minutes leads to the formation of enough acid to damage the teeth.

The verdict

Whichever way we look at the issue, the verdict is clear: starch is better than sugar. Therefore, we should consume our carbohydrates as much as possible in the form of starch, and as little as we can in the form of sugar.

Dietary fibre

Dietary fibre includes a large family of heterogenous chemical entities, but the head of the family, cellulose, is a close cousin of carbohydrates. Two characteristics are common to all members of the fibre family—one, that they occur only in plant foods; and two, that they cannot be digested by any of the juices in our stomach or intestines. However, some members of the family can be digested (rather, fermented) by germs that normally reside in our large intestine. Fermentation is associated with production of gases; the gases so produced announce their departure from the body as flatus. Besides embarrassing us by turning us into the source of unwanted noise and odour, what else does fibre do? Since fibre is not digested, it does not contribute to energy intake. But still we need fibre, and we need lots of it. Refined foods (such as white rice and refined wheat flour or maida) have contributed to the emergence of the diseases of modern civilization, such as piles, varicose veins, obesity, diabetes, heart disease and intestinal cancer.

Why do we need fibre?

Since fibre does not get digested, it is just passed on from the stomach to the small intestine, and from the small intestine to the large intestine. One of the properties of fibre is that it soaks water, swells up and forms a viscous mass. The mass adds bulk to the contents of the large intestine and does not let them become dry or hard. That is how fibre prevents constipation. Fibre not only facilitates the frequent passage of stool, it also makes the stool soft. Constipation is not just a minor inconvenience. Chronic constipation is the mother of piles and varicose veins. Ispaghula husk (isabgol) is a concentrated source of fibre. If you soak a spoon of isabgol in water for a few minutes, it grows in volume and forms a viscous gel. That is why isabgol can help treat constipation.

Besides preventing constipation, fibre is now known to have important metabolic consequences. It improves glucose tolerance and reduces blood cholesterol. These actions of fibre make it important for the prevention and management of diabetes and coronary heart disease.

How can we get enough fibre?

Fibre is plentiful in unrefined grains, fruits and vegetables. To get enough fibre, we should consume grains which have their husk (seed coat) intact. For example, brown bread is better in this respect than white bread, and brown rice (or parboiled rice, sela chawal) is better than white rice. Coarse grains, such as barley (jau), oat and buckwheat (kuttoo) are also good sources of fibre. For making chapattis, the more coarse, i.e. with more bran, the atta, the better. Among the dals, those with the husk intact are preferable to those from which the husk has been removed. For example, sabut moong is better than dhuli moong. Among fruits and vegetables, green leafy vegetables are preferable as sources of dietary fibre. Incidentally, whole grains (those with the husk intact) and green leafy vegetables are also good sources of vitamins and minerals. The husks of grains have much more vitamins and minerals than the interiors of the grains.

There is a popular misconception that if one consumes enough fruits and vegetables, fibre intake will take care of itself. This is erroneous for a variety of reasons. First, 80 per cent of the weight of most fruits and vegetables is made up of water. All the remaining constituents are packed in less than 20 per cent, and therefore, there is not much scope for getting adequate fibre from only fruits and vegetables. Second, eating enough fruits and vegetables means having about five hundred grams of these (or five moderate helpings), and very few of us have that much. Finally, the type of fibre found in fruits and vegetables is qualitatively different from that in cereals and pulses. The fibres from these two sources have somewhat distinct functions. Therefore, getting fibre from both is important. In short, even if we consume enough fruits and vegetables (about five hundred grams per day), we should eat fibre-rich coarse (unrefined) food grains. Because of the large amount of grains we consume, they are potentially the major source of fibre in our diet. If we consume the right type of grains, they will give us much more fibre than fruits and vegetables. Without the right grains, fruits and vegetables cannot ordinarily meet our fibre requirements.

Frequently Asked Questions

How much sugar do we need?

We do not need sugar at all.* Human beings have survived for thousands of years before sugar was manufactured. However, we may take small quantities of sugar if we want to. The upper limit is quite generous: about 10 per cent of the energy intake. Thus, if a person has 2,000 Calories per day, he may obtain 200 Calories from sugar. Since sugar gives 4 Calories per gram, 200 Calories would come from 50 grams of sugar. One level teaspoon of sugar has about 5 grams of sugar. Thus, a person may

*There is a big difference between 'We *do not need* sugar at all' and 'We *should not consume* sugar at all'.

take up to ten teaspoons of sugar per day. People who consume a lot of tea, coffee, cold drinks, sweets, cake and ice cream regularly may end up taking more than 100 grams of sugar per day, which is definitely undesirable. In short, the less sugar one consumes, the better, but under no circumstances should a person have more than 50 grams of sugar in a day.

Why should a person suffering from constipation take no laxatives?

Contrary to common belief, laxatives do not cure constipation. Laxatives empty out a much longer length of the large intestine than is normal during defecation. The result is that after a laxative-induced motion, it takes time (maybe two days or more) for the large intestine to fill up enough to create an urge for defecation. During these two days, the person may get all the more convinced that he has very obstinate constipation. If he does not have the patience to wait for two to three days, he takes another dose of laxative. The laxative leads to a motion all right, but at the expense of emptying too much of the bowels. The result is another bout of constipation until enough fecal matter has collected. Thus, the laxative itself becomes the cause of constipation.

However, a person may take isabgol for constipation. Isabgol is not a laxative. It is a dietary supplement. It facilitates passing motion by making the stool bulkier and softer.

How might refrigerated food produce more flatus than freshly cooked food?

Refrigeration converts a small part of the starch present in foods into 'resistant starch'. Resistant starch cannot be digested by the human digestive juices, but can be fermented by the germs residing in the large intestine. Thus, resistant starch behaves like the fermentable fraction of dietary fibre, and leads to flatulence.

How can we reduce flatulence?

Flatulence may be reduced by:
- (a) Avoiding certain beans, especially kidney beans (rajma), chickpeas (chane) and black gram (urad).
- (b) Instead of the above beans, having mung beans (moong) or lentils (masoor).
- (c) Increasing the consumption of ginger (adrak/saunth), omum (ajwain), aniseed (saunf) and asafoetida (hing).
- (d) Increasing the consumption of curd.
- (e) Avoiding milk, if it increases flatulence.
- (f) Avoiding high fat foods.
- (g) Avoiding non-vegetarian food.

SUMMARY

1. In a good diet, about 70 per cent of the energy comes from carbohydrates.
2. Dietary carbohydrates are either starches (complex carbohydrates) or sugars (simple carbohydrates).

3. We get most of our carbohydrates from cereals and pulses.
4. Carbohydrates give 4 Calories per gram.
5. Starch is preferable to sugar because:

    (a) Starchy foods also have other nutrients whereas sugar is 100 per cent carbohydrate.
    (b) After eating sugar, the blood sugar level rises faster and to a higher peak than after consuming the same amount of carbohydrates in the form of a starchy food.
    (c) Sugar promotes overeating.
    (d) Sugar-containing foods carry a high risk of giving us dental cavities.

6. Although dietary fibre is not digested, we need it because:

    (a) It prevents constipation and its sequelae such as piles and varicose veins.
    (b) It helps prevent weight gain, diabetes, heart disease and intestinal cancer.

7. In order to get enough fibre, we should consume unrefined cereals and pulses, coarse grains, fruits and vegetables.

3
The Dethroned King

Vanity dies hard; in some obstinate cases it outlives the man.

ROBERT LOUIS STEVENSON

Proteins are often placed on a pedestal for reasons that have not stood the test of time. We do need some amount of protein, but taking more than what we need is not necessarily better. Moreover, the amount of protein that we need is easy to obtain from an ordinary traditional Indian diet.

How much protein do we need?

A healthy adult needs about 1 gram of protein per day for each kilogram of body weight. Thus, a 60 kg adult needs 60 g protein per day. Another way to express the protein requirement is as a fraction of the total energy requirement. To understand this, it is important to know that 1 gram of protein gives us 4 Calories. Although protein may be used by the body not for getting energy but for building the body (i.e. not as fuel but as construction material), it is convenient in the present context to think of protein in terms of the energy it can possibly give us. Coming back to our protein requirement, it is 10 per cent of our total energy intake. Suppose a moderately active, 60 kg person needs 2,400 Calories per day. This person will need 10 per cent of 2,400 Calories, i.e. 240 Calories from protein. To get 4 Calories, we have to take 1 g of protein. Hence, to get 240 Calories from protein, the person should take 60 g of protein per day. Thus, the protein requirement works out to be about the same figure, no matter how we calculate it.

How can we obtain the protein?

It comes as a surprise to most people that the single largest source of protein in the Indian diet are the cereals, and that there is nothing wrong with this. A typical cereal, such as wheat or rice, has protein to the tune of about 10 per cent of its weight (Fig. 3.1). Thus, if a person eats 500 g of any cereal per day, it gives him 50 g of protein. Pulses, such as green gram or red gram, have 20 per cent protein, which is about double as compared to cereals, but we take hardly 100 g of a pulse (or dal) per day. If we do that, it would give us another 20 g of protein. Thus, 500 g of a cereal and 100 g of a pulse give us about 70 g of protein, and that is more than enough for most people.

Of course, there are other sources of protein in our diet, such as milk, cheese, curd (or yogurt), egg and meat. These foods may have a place in the diet, but we do not have to depend upon them for satisfying our protein requirement.

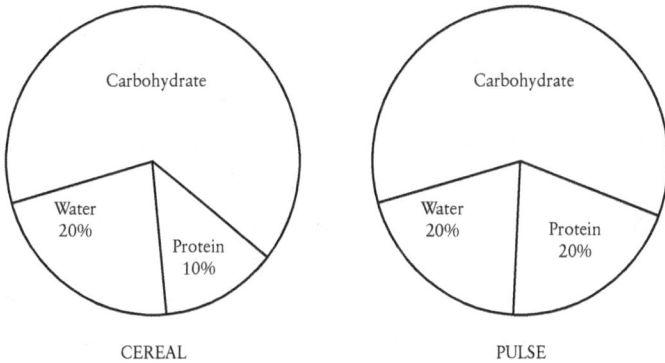

Fig. 3.1. Approximate composition of a typical cereal and pulse. Note that both have plenty of carbohydrate (starch). Further, cereals also have protein. In fact, cereals are the single largest source of protein in the Indian diet.

How about quality?

Just as all carbohydrates are not alike, all proteins are also not alike. In case of proteins, the difference resides in their 'quality'. The quality of a protein refers to how good it is as food. For understanding the concept of 'protein quality', it is necessary to go into a bit of their chemistry.*

---

*If you have an aversion to chemistry, you may skip the next paragraph.

Protein molecules are large molecules. The building blocks of protein molecules are called amino acids. There are twenty different amino acids found in human proteins. The body has to keep manufacturing protein continuously to replace wear and tear, and in case of children, also for growth. This would not be a problem if the body could manufacture amino acids from some readily available raw materials. In fact, the body can manufacture ten amino acids in this way. But the other ten amino acids have to be supplied ready-made to the body, from food. During digestion, dietary protein is dismantled into its constituent amino acids. Some of the amino acids that food proteins yield are those which the body can also manufacture, while others are those which the body cannot manufacture. The amino acids which the body cannot manufacture are called essential amino acids (EAA)—they are called 'essential' because it is essential to obtain them from dietary protein. It is not enough to get all the EAAs from food. Ideally, dietary protein should supply individual EAAs in the same proportion as is required for manufacturing body proteins. The proportion of individual EAA in proteins varies in different living organisms. Similar organisms have similar proteins. Man being more similar to animals than plants, human proteins are more like animal proteins than plant proteins. Hence, the proportion of EAA in animal proteins is similar to that in human proteins, but the proportion of EAA in plant proteins is quite different. This is what is meant by saying that animal proteins are good quality proteins, while plant proteins are poor in quality. However, individual plant proteins are also not exactly alike in this respect. The EAA whose level is relatively the lowest in the protein in relation to what it should be from the point of view of human dietary requirements, is called the limiting amino acid. The limiting amino acid in different plant proteins is not the same. Hence, plant proteins can be combined in our diet in such a way that the deficiency of an EAA in one plant protein is made up by another plant protein. The classical combination of this type is the cereal–pulse combination. Cereals are deficient in the EAA called lysine, whereas pulses are deficient in the EAA called methionine. In a cereal–pulse combination, the lysine deficiency of the cereal is made up by the pulse, and the methionine deficiency of the pulse is made up by the cereal.

In short*, although cereal protein is poor in quality, and so is pulse protein, when the two are combined, we get good quality protein. This is not just a theoretical expectation: studies have confirmed that growth is just as good on a cereal–pulse combination as on animal protein. Milk and milk products are the only sources of animal protein available to vegetarians. Non-vegetarians may also get animal protein from egg, fish or meat.

---

*If you decided to skip the chemistry behind protein quality, you may start from here.

WHY GO VEG?

There is a worldwide wave driving people towards vegetarian diets. There are at least three reasons for going vegetarian.

First, vegetarian diets are not only adequate and satisfactory, they are also more healthy than non-vegetarian diets. Non-vegetarian diets contribute to the risk of getting heart disease, appendicitis, diverticulitis, osteoporosis and cancer of the large intestine. In contrast, only plant foods have the protective factors currently grouped under phytochemicals, which reduce the risk for getting heart disease, diabetes, infections and cancer (See Chapter 7).

Second, vegetarian diets are more ethical. No sensitive human being eats meat without, at least sometimes, feeling a sense of guilt. This sense of uneasiness has nothing to do with religion. No religion compels a person to eat meat; no religion prevents a person from giving up meat.

Third, vegetarian diets are more eco-friendly. In the ultimate analysis, meat also originates in plants because the animals that give us meat themselves eat grass. However, the process of converting plant material into meat is very inefficient. It has been estimated that it takes 30 kg of plant protein for us to get 1 kg of animal protein. More than 90 per cent of the agricultural land in the United States is used for growing grass for animals destined to die in slaughterhouses. If people stop eating meat, all this land would be available for growing food for human consumption. If every person in the world turns vegetarian, the problem of world hunger can be wiped out in one stroke. Further, the waste gases emitted by animals belonging to the meat industry, the equipment for processing and storage used by the meat industry, transportation of meat, etc. contribute to global warming. A UN report published in 2006 has estimated that the contribution of the meat industry to global warming exceeds that of all the SUVs, ships and aeroplanes of the world put together. If everybody turns vegetarian, we can therefore forget about the dangers of global warming for a long time to come. Thus, vegetarianism is no longer an issue that revolves around individual choice for the sake of good health or for ethical reasons. Vegetarian diets give us the best chance of surviving on a planet fast getting depleted and poisoned by the activities associated with modern civilization.

What about children?

We have seen above that a cereal–pulse combination can supply all the protein that an adult needs. Does that also apply to children? Let us examine this issue by considering the case of a child weighing 10 kg. This child would need 2 g/kg body weight of dietary protein everyday, which is, in a way, twice as much as an adult needs. However, let us consider the issue further. The 20 g of protein that this child may take gives him 80 Calories. The total daily energy requirement of this child is 100 Calories/kg body weight, i.e. 1,000 Calories. The 80 Calories from protein constitute only 8 per cent of the 1,000 Calories that the child consumes. Looked at this way, the child needs slightly less protein than an adult. Thus, the child needs more protein or less protein than an adult, depending on how we express it. This funny paradox is not difficult to explain (Table 3.1). The child needs not only more protein, but also more energy than an adult on a 'per kg body weight' basis. Therefore, the fraction of the total energy intake that needs to come from protein remains essentially constant at about 10 per cent throughout one's life. The implications of this fraction remaining constant are important: foods which provide about 10 per cent of their energy content through protein can meet the protein requirement of all age groups, provided such foods are the staple diet. Cereals have 10 per cent protein, and pulses have 20 per cent protein. Therefore, more than 10 per cent of the energy that a cereal–pulse mixture gives will come from protein. Thus, a cereal–pulse mixture, which is the backbone of an Indian diet, meets this important requirement. Further, a mixture of cereal and pulse protein is also good in quality. Hence, a diet in which the staple foods are cereals and pulses can meet the protein requirements of children as well as adults, both in terms of quantity as well as quality. This is the basis of the dictum that if energy intake is adequate, protein intake will take care of itself.

Table 3.1. Energy and protein requirements of a child and an adult

	Body weight	Protein requirement	Protein Calories	Energy requirement	Protein Calories (per cent)
Child	10 kg	2 g/kg, i.e. 20 g	20x4 = 80	100 Cal/kg i.e. 1,000 Cal	80/1000 = 8 per cent
Adult	50 kg	1 g/kg, i.e. 50 g	50x4 = 200	40 Cal/kg i.e. 2,000 Cal	200/2000 = 10 per cent

Closing thoughts

The foods that form the backbone of the ordinary Indian diet are cereals and pulses. These two foods together can meet the protein needs of children as well as adults. The quality of protein obtained from a cereal–pulse mixture is also satisfactory. Hence, there is normally no justification for any exotic or expensive sources of protein. High protein foods may be necessary under some conditions, such as certain diseases; in those situations, it is best to follow a doctor's advice.

Frequently Asked Questions

Can too much protein in the diet be harmful?

Yes, there is considerable evidence that taking far more protein than necessary can be harmful. One, it increases the urinary loss of calcium. Therefore, it increases the dietary requirement of calcium. Hence, it can increase the risk of osteoporosis. By increasing the urinary concentration of calcium, high protein diets may also add to the risk of urinary stones. Two, proteins metabolized to form urea. Urea has to be removed from the body by the kidneys. Therefore, taking too much protein overloads the kidneys. There are many other good and bad effects that have been attributed to high protein diets. But the plain truth is that we need exactly the amount of protein that is readily available from a cereal–pulse mixture. More protein than that is unnecessary. Even if the extra protein does not do us any significant harm, it will be used up by the body as fuel. Using protein as fuel instead of carbohydrate is like burning furniture instead of firewood to cook food.

What are the special benefits of soya bean?

Soya bean has a unique composition—high protein (about 40 per cent) and high fat (about 20 per cent)—but no special benefits. It is an acceptable food, but its higher protein content is not essential for meeting our protein needs. There are several other potential benefits that have been attributed to it in an attempt to popularize it. One, it has n-3 PUFA (See Chapter 4). But, for n-3 PUFA, it makes more sense to depend on soya bean oil or mustard oil, rather than use the soya bean itself. Two, it has phytochemicals which have effects similar to the female hormone estrogen. A weak estrogenic effect is not limited to soya bean: it is there in many plant foods (See Chapter 7). Three, it may reduce blood cholesterol levels. But this effect is weak. Moreover, many other plant foods, especially high-fibre foods, have this effect. Finally, blood cholesterol is affected by a large number of lifestyle factors, of which nutrition is only one, and within nutrition, soya bean is just one food; and that too, one that is unlikely to be consumed predictably in significant amounts on a regular basis by an average Indian. Finally, blood cholesterol is only one of the several modifiable risk factors for heart disease. Therefore, it makes no sense to highlight soya bean as that single miracle food that will protect us from heart disease.

SUMMARY

1. Healthy children, as well as adults, need about 10 per cent of their energy intake in the form of protein.

2. Protein requirements of all age groups can be met satisfactorily by a diet in which the staple food is a mixture of cereals and pulses.

3. Although cereal and pulse proteins individually are of poor quality, their combination yields protein of good quality. This happens because the deficiency in cereal protein is made up by pulse protein, and the deficiency in pulse protein is made up by cereal protein.

4. Animal foods are not essential for good health. In fact, vegetarian diets are healthier, more eco-friendly and ethically more sound than non-vegetarian diets.

5. A cereal–pulse combination can take care of the protein requirement of healthy children as well as adults. Therefore, exotic and expensive foods having high concentrations of protein are not normally necessary.

4
Densely Packed

Everyone is needed; nobody is needed much.

RALPH WALDO EMERSON

After carbohydrates and proteins, we come to the third and last nutrient that also gives energy, namely, fat. Fats are a concentrated source of energy. In contrast with carbohydrates and proteins, which give 4 Calories per gram, each gram of fat gives 9 Calories.

How much?

We do need a small amount of essential fats, but that amount is available to us through cereals, pulses and vegetables. Since these fats enter the diet imperceptibly, they are collectively called invisible fat. In addition, we consume visible fat in the form of oils, butter and ghee. It is currently recommended that not more than 30 per cent of our energy intake should come from fats. This is not really a hardship for Indians, because barring rich food consumed during festivals and celebrations, Indian diets seldom provide more fat than that.

Let us assume that about 5 per cent of the energy intake comes from invisible fat, and a person wants to consume only 15 per cent more of the energy intake in the form of visible fat. If the person's energy intake is 2,000 Calories per day, it comes to 300 Calories in the form of visible fat. Since each gram of fat gives 9 Calories, to get these 300 Calories, the person should take about 33 grams of fat everyday, which comes to 990 grams of fat a month. In short, if a person's visible fat intake is 1 kilo per month, visible fat will provide him about 15 per cent of the energy intake. If we add to that the contribution of the invisible fat, his fat energy will be about 20 per cent of the total energy intake; certainly less than the permissible 30 per cent. Thus, as a rule of thumb, a family of five should consume not more than one 5 kg container of oil.

However, the lifestyle of many families is such that further restriction may be necessary. If the family eats a lot of snacks and meals at parties and in restaurants, consumes butter or ghee in addition to the oil used as the cooking medium and also consumes a significant quantity of nuts*, the permissible limit for the cooking medium has to be brought down. Therefore, many physicians advise consuming less than half a kilo of the cooking medium per person per month.

---

*Nuts are high-fat foods.

Which fats?

Research on the relationship between dietary fat and heart disease over the last fifty years has been the basis of the recommendations regarding desirable and undesirable dietary fats. But unfortunately, the recommendations have been changing, as the research itself has evolved and matured. This has resulted in considerable confusion because while recommendations can be revised with the stroke of a pen (or, as we now say, the click of a mouse), deeply ingrained ideas have a tendency to persist.

To understand the research and recommendations, it is necessary to go into some technicalities*. What distinguishes one dietary fat from another is the type of fatty acids it contains. There are three broad categories of fatty acids (FA): saturated, monounsaturated and polyunsaturated (SFA, MUFA and PUFA respectively). PUFA is further divided into two types: n-3 PUFA and n-6 PUFA. The same dietary fat may have more than one type of fatty acids, but one type may dominate the composition. Traditionally, people have consumed diets that provide a mixture of all types of fatty acids. Research done in the 1950s and 1960s indicated that (a) high levels of blood cholesterol are associated with a high risk for heart disease; and (b) SFA raises blood cholesterol whereas PUFA lowers the blood cholesterol levels†. MUFA

---

*If you don't want to read about the technicalities, you may skip this paragraph.
†Cholesterol will be discussed in greater detail a little later in the chapter.

is relatively neutral in its effects on blood cholesterol. On the basis of this research, it was concluded that the lower the blood cholesterol, the better; and therefore, more the PUFA and less the SFA in the diet, the better. Therefore, in India, people were advised to give up butter and ghee (which have about two-thirds SFA and one-third MUFA), and to switch over to oils such as corn oil, sesame oil, sunflower oil, safflower oil and cottonseed oil (which are almost entirely n-6 PUFA). This was standard advice for more than three decades, and has not died down even today. While the research on which these recommendations were based is still valid, it had overlooked many finer points which were brought out by subsequent research. First, high blood cholesterol is just one of the several risk factors for heart disease. Second, very low levels of blood cholesterol also carry some health risks. Third, high PUFA diets may weaken the immune system, which may increase the risk for several diseases, including heart disease. And finally, a very high n-6 to n-3 PUFA ratio in the diet increases the tendency of the blood to clot and induces inflammation of the walls of arteries—both these factors may increase the risk for heart disease, the very reason for which high n-6 PUFA diets were recommended in the first place! One could go on about the harmful effects of lopsided high n-6 PUFA intake, but to cut a long story short, by the 1990s, research had reached a stage that warranted a revision in the recommendations regarding fat intake. The current recommendation is that the dietary fat should have approximately equal quantities of SFA, MUFA and PUFA, and that the n-6 to n-3 PUFA ratio should preferably be 5 or less.

What does the current advice mean in terms of selection of oils and fats*? It means that the best oils for cooking are mustard oil and soya bean oil, because these are the only ones among the oils commonly available in India that have SFA, MUFA, n-3 PUFA and also n-6 PUFA. The supply of n-3 PUFA is an important limiting factor. We may get SFA and MUFA from butter, ghee or palm oil; and n-6 PUFA from corn oil or sunflower oil; but none of these is a good source of n-3 PUFA. Therefore, a simple and convenient option is to adopt mustard oil or soya bean oil (or both) as the principal cooking medium, and supplement it with a small quantity of butter and ghee to bring the SFA and MUFA to the same level as the PUFA. Now, let us examine a few other oils to see why some other, more glamorous options might not be necessarily better.

Olive oil

Olive oil is a high-MUFA oil. Therefore, in order to get SFA and PUFA, it will have to be supplemented with other appropriate oils. Secondly, its 'smoking point' is low, or to put it simply, olive oil does not stand heating well. Therefore it is not very suitable for cooking. But, as dressing for salads, olive oil is acceptable. However, olive oil is not essential for staying healthy.

---

*If you decided to skip the technical discussion, you may resume reading from here.

Rice bran oil

Rice bran oil is similar to sunflower oil and corn oil in having n-6 PUFA but no n-3 PUFA. However, its n-6 PUFA is accompanied by a significant amount of MUFA, which makes it similar to a blend of sunflower or corn oil with olive oil.

Groundnut oil

Groundnut oil has a variety of fatty acids. In contrast to sunflower oil and corn oil, which have only n-6 PUFA, groundnut oil also has in addition a small but significant quantity of SFA and MUFA. But groundnut oil also has no n-3 PUFA.

Rapeseed oil

Rapeseed oil has a composition similar to mustard oil. It has decent amounts of SFA, MUFA, n-6 PUFA and n-3 PUFA, and may be used for cooking. However, there is some reservation about it because of its high erucic acid content.

Canola oil

Canola oil is a low erucic acid variant of rapeseed oil, and is therefore acceptable as the principal cooking medium. Theoretically, it can replace mustard oil or rapeseed oil, but it is still controversial whether the replacement is necessary. Canola oil is now available in India, and its price is also comparable to that of other refined oils.

Coconut oil

Coconut oil is an exception among vegetable oils as it has very high levels of SFA. That is why, like the SFA-rich butter and ghee, coconut oil also becomes solid in winters. Since SFA, in general, raises blood cholesterol, coconut oil may also be expected to do so but it does not. This paradox seems to occur because all SFAs are not alike. The SFA in coconut oil is mainly of the medium-chain type (MCFA).* MCFA does not raise serum cholesterol, and coconut oil may even be beneficial because of its antioxidant, immuno-enhancing, and anti-infective activity. People in Kerala (India), Sri Lanka and several other tropical countries have used coconut oil as the principal cooking medium for several generations. These populations neither have a tendency towards high cholesterol levels, nor a high prevalence of heart disease attributable to the oil they consume. This natural experiment, which has been going on for centuries, further supports the suitability of coconut oil as a primary source of dietary fat, especially for those who have adapted to it over several generations.

---

*'Medium chain' refers to the length of the carbon chain in the molecules of the fatty acid. Medium chain fats are easier to digest and absorb, and possibly that is why they act as sources of quickly available energy rather than lead to metabolic effects such as high blood cholesterol levels. For the same reason, when digestion is weak or impaired, coconut oil is the easiest to digest.

Hydrogenated vegetable oils

Hydrogenation is an artificial process that converts the PUFA in vegetable oils into SFA. The conversion also imparts the oils the solidity and stability of SFA-rich fats like butter and ghee. But hydrogenation also generates trans fatty acids, which are associated with increase in the risk for heart disease. That is an additional reason why hydrogenated vegetable oils should not be used for cooking. However, hydrogenated oils are commonly used in biscuits, fried potato chips and namkeens because of their long shelf-life. Therefore, the intake of these foods should be restricted in order to reduce the trans fatty acid intake. Margarine is made by partial hydrogenation of vegetable oils. Since hydrogenation is incomplete, it is not as hard as fully hydrogenated oils. But since some hydrogenation has taken place, margarine is not liquid like oils either. In short, margarine is soft like butter. But margarine may also have trans fatty acids, and therefore should be avoided.

Flaxseed oil

Flaxseed oil is not a cooking medium. It is a nutritional supplement that provides n-3 PUFA. If the dietary fat is judiciously chosen, this supplement is not required. However, if it has to be taken, its quantity should be less than 15 grams per day. Further, flaxseed oil interacts dangerously with a wide variety of commonly used drugs such as pain-killers, lipid-lowering drugs and many of the drugs used in the treatment of high blood pressure, heart disease and diabetes. Therefore, those on any long-term medication should consult their physician before taking a flaxseed oil supplement.

Fish oil

Fish oil is also not a cooking medium but a nutritional supplement that provides n-3 PUFA; cod liver oil also has vitamins A and D. As a supplement, 1 gram of fish oil is comparable to about 7 grams of flaxseed oil. Fish oil supplements also need the same precautions as flaxseed oil supplements.

Cholesterol

The much-maligned cholesterol is a close cousin of fats. Cholesterol is not a poison. It is a normal constituent of the body, and also of the diet. However, excess of everything is bad, and so is that of cholesterol. The excess may be in the diet or in the body, and the two may be related by cause and effect.

Levels of cholesterol in the blood should normally be less than 200 mg/dL. Higher levels than that are associated with heart disease. However, high cholesterol level is only one among several risk factors for heart disease. Moreover, dietary cholesterol is only one of the dietary factors that affect blood cholesterol. Being overweight, sedentary lifestyle, smoking and mental stress are the factors other than diet that raise blood cholesterol. Further, blood cholesterol has a few factions. Of these, only high levels of LDL cholesterol raise the risk for heart disease; it is desirable to maintain LDL levels below 100 mg/dL. In contrast, high levels of HDL cholesterol reduce the risk of heart disease; the desirable HDL level is above 60 mg/dL.*

Cholesterol in the body may come from the diet or may be manufactured in the body. The body has a mechanism for matching the supply of cholesterol with its requirement. If the diet has more cholesterol, the body manufactures less cholesterol; if the diet has less cholesterol, the body manufactures more; and if the diet has no cholesterol, the body manufactures all the cholesterol that it needs. However, this regulatory mechanism has its limits. It is possible to take so much cholesterol in the diet that this mechanism is overwhelmed, and the breakdown of the mechanism is reflected in high blood cholesterol. The amount of dietary cholesterol that will overwhelm the mechanism varies with individuals. About one-third of the population is rather sensitive, and responds to even modest amounts of dietary cholesterol with a marked rise in blood cholesterol. Such persons are called hyper-responders.

It has been found that those who are not hyper-responders are able to maintain normal blood cholesterol levels if their dietary cholesterol is less than 300 mg per day. For vegetarians, it is very easy to stay within this limit because no plant food contains any cholesterol. For them, the only sources of cholesterol are milk and milk products. These sources will generally give a person about 50 mg of cholesterol in a day. Among the commonly

---

*An easy way to remember it is: L for lousy, H for healthy.

consumed non-vegetarian foods, egg is the richest source of cholesterol. One egg contains 250 mg of cholesterol. All the cholesterol in the egg is in the yellow part; the white of the egg contains no cholesterol. Most non-vegetarian Indians generally consume only small amounts of meat, and that too, not everyday. Therefore, having one egg per day still leaves the cholesterol intake of most Indians within the permissible limit of 300 mg per day. However, that will not apply to hyper-responders, and their number is not negligible. The best way to find out if one is a hyper-responder is to do a short experiment on oneself. Have no eggs for a month. Get blood cholesterol level tested. Eat one egg a day for a month. Get blood cholesterol level tested again. If the second blood cholesterol level is significantly higher, and above the normal range, the person is a hyper-responder. This experiment is required only if a person wants to eat eggs. Strict vegetarians can forget about how much cholesterol they are taking—they will never be able to exceed their limit even if they are hyper-responders.

No Plant Food Contains Cholesterol

Mustard oil contains no cholesterol

Soya bean oil contains no cholesterol

Groundnut oil contains no cholesterol

Coconut oil contains no cholesterol

Almonds contain no cholesterol

Walnuts contain no cholesterol

Cashew nuts contain no cholesterol

Because all the above foods are plant foods

In short, a healthy person who is not at high risk of getting heart disease, has normal blood cholesterol levels and is not a hyper-responder, may take up to 300 mg of cholesterol per day. In the context of an Indian diet, this will usually allow him to have up to one egg per day. However, such a person will not suffer from any deficiency if he takes less cholesterol than that, or even no cholesterol at all. Those who have a hereditary tendency towards high cholesterol levels, are hyper-responders or have heart disease should not consume eggs, and consult a physician for advice on lifestyle modification.

Table 4.1 Cholesterol Content of Foods

Food	Cholesterol Content (approx.)
Mutton, chicken, fish	100 mg/100 g
Liver, kidney	300 mg/100 g
Brain	2000 mg/100 g
Egg, one	250 mg
Milk, whole	40 mg/glass
Ice cream	50 mg/small cup
Fish oils	500 mg/100 g
Butter	200 mg/100 g
Ghee	200 mg/100 g
All vegetable oils	0 mg/100 g
All nuts	0 mg/100 g

Conclusion

As in many other areas of nutrition, science has travelled full circle too in relation to fats. Traditional oils, such as mustard oil and coconut oil, are back. Butter and ghee are no longer taboo. However, moderation continues to be the golden rule. All fats give 9 Calories per gram. Therefore, too much of any fat is likely to lead to weight gain. Also, excess of any fat may raise the blood cholesterol level; the difference may be only that of degree. On the other hand, moderate quantities of well-selected fats within the framework of a balanced diet and a healthy lifestyle are perfectly acceptable.

Frequently Asked Questions

Are blends of different oils acceptable?

Yes, blends are acceptable, but they offer a significant advantage over single oils only if their constituents have been judiciously chosen. A partial survey of cooking oils available in the market discovered the following blends:

- Soya bean oil (80 per cent) + sunflower oil (20 per cent): It is difficult to understand how diluting soya bean oil with sunflower oil would help. Because of sunflower oil being very rich in n-6 PUFA and having no n-3 PUFA, the blend has an n-3:n-6 ratio of 1:11, which is much lower than the recommended 1:5. Soya bean oil alone would be better, with an n-3:n-6 ratio of 1:7.8.

- Rice bran oil (80 per cent) + sunflower oil (20 per cent): It is, again, difficult to understand how diluting rice bran oil with sunflower oil would help. Rice bran oil (RBO) is also not perfect. The good thing about RBO is its high MUFA content. But like most of the other vegetable oils, RBO also has no n-3 PUFA. Mixing two oils, neither of them having n-3 PUFA, makes no scientific sense.

- Safflower (kardi) oil + rice bran oil (percentages not specified): Yet again, it is difficult to understand how diluting safflower oil with RBO would help. Once again, neither of the oils in the blend has n-3 PUFA. The point highlighted on the container is that the oil contains orynzol, which lowers blood cholesterol. Orynzol is a constituent of RBO. But blood cholesterol is affected by such a large number of dietary and non-dietary lifestyle factors that a little bit of orynzol cannot make a big difference.

In short, none of the above blends makes scientific sense. Compared to these blends, it would be much better to stick to soya bean oil, mustard oil or canola oil. Many of the oils available have been fortified with vitamins A, D and E, which is acceptable, and may be particularly helpful in supplementing the vitamin D intake of vegetarians (see also Chapters 5 and 8).

Are zero cholesterol oils preferable to other oils?

Almost all oils used in cooking are vegetable oils. They are all 'zero cholesterol' oils because no food of plant origin contains any cholesterol. Therefore, when an advertisement says that a particular brand of oil is zero cholesterol, it is telling the truth, but not the whole truth. That oil is, of course, zero cholesterol, but so are all the other vegetable oils. Hence, the oil that we use does not affect *dietary* cholesterol. How the oil affects *blood* cholesterol is another issue, and that has already been discussed in the chapter at considerable length.

How do refined oils differ from unrefined oils, and do these differences have any important implications?

Unrefined oils are obtained by treating oilseeds with the cold-pressed or expeller-pressed methods. These are relatively crude and ancient methods. What we get by these methods is not just the oil but also a few other substances in the oilseed, and therefore the oil is unrefined. Unrefined oils have a strong odour, and do not stand high temperatures well. But many of the additional substances that they contain may have beneficial effects, e.g. unrefined palm oil has carotenes, and many unrefined vegetable oils have vitamin E, which is not only nutritionally important but also prolongs the shelf-life of the oil.

Refined oils are obtained by solvent-extraction, and the process involves heating the oil to high temperatures.

As a result, vitamin E is lost, and the shelf-life of refined oils has to be extended by using preservatives. Other than the oil, the refined oils contain no other substance in significant amount. They are bleached, and are therefore nearly colourless; they are deodorized, and are therefore odourless; they tolerate heat well, and are therefore suitable also for deep frying. Hence, refined oils are generally more suitable for cooking.

How does heating affect the effects of an oil?

Heating changes the oil physically and chemically. Physically, the viscosity of the oil is altered. Chemically, it may acquire some carcinogenic substances. This is more likely if the oil also contains some food particles, which may get burnt to produce carcinogens. Therefore, oil left over after frying should not be used repeatedly. Repeated cycles of frying makes the oil more harmful. Oil left over after one cycle of frying should be finished by adding to a vegetable or dal. Among the commonly used vegetable oils, the one that stands heat the best is coconut oil.

What are the important sources of n-3 PUFA in the diet?

Among the common cooking media, mustard oil and soya bean oil are the only ones which have n-3 PUFA. Another valuable source of n-3 PUFA in the diet is the invisible fat present in beans and green leafy vegetables. Non-vegetarians can also get n-3 PUFA from fish and fish oil supplements. A currently popular supplement that supplies n-3 PUFA is flaxseed oil.

How does ghee differ from butter in terms of its health effects?

Ghee has no water. Therefore, its calorific value is higher, and shelf-life longer than that of butter. It withstands high temperatures extremely well, and is therefore suitable for deep frying.

What are the risks associated with very low blood cholesterol levels?

There are some reports suggesting that very low total blood cholesterol levels are associated with depression and cancer. But there is still no consensus on how low is too low.

What are triglycerides, and what are the risks associated with high blood triglyceride levels?

Triglycerides are fats. All the dietary fats and oils are, chemically, triglycerides. We have triglycerides in our bodies. We also have triglycerides circulating in our blood. The normal blood triglyceride level is less than 150 mg/dL. Higher levels than that are associated with increase in the risk of heart disease. Blood triglycerides may rise above the desirable level due to an unhealthy lifestyle, particularly lack of physical activity, eating too much, eating an unhealthy diet, smoking and drinking. Among dietary factors, refined carbohydrates (e.g. sugar, maida and white rice) are particularly associated with high triglyceride levels.

SUMMARY

1. Fats are a concentrated source of energy. In contrast to carbohydrates and proteins, which give 4 Calories per gram, each gram of fat gives 9 Calories.

2. Our diet contains some invisible fat that we get from grains, fruits and vegetables; and some visible fat that we get from oils, butter and ghee.

3. Not more than 30 per cent of our energy intake should come from fats. The consumption of visible fats should be less than 1 kg per month for an adult.

4. The best cooking oils are mustard oil and soya bean oil, because these oils have SFA, MUFA, n-3 PUFA and also n-6 PUFA.

5. No food of plant origin contains cholesterol.

6. Moderation in the intake of fats is important because all fats give 9 Calories per gram. Therefore, too much of *any* fat is likely to lead to excess weight. Also, too much of any fat and being overweight may raise the blood cholesterol level. On the other hand, moderate quantities of judiciously chosen fats within the framework of a balanced diet and healthy lifestyle are perfectly acceptable.

5
Small Is Beautiful

The great and the little have need of one another.

THOMAS FULLER

To make fire, we need not only fuel, but also a matchstick. Although the matchstick is small in size as compared to the huge amount of fuel required, it is indispensable. Similarly, in our diet we need certain nutrients in very small amounts, without which the large amounts of carbohydrate, protein and fat that we take cannot be properly utilized. The traditional nutrients in this category are vitamins and minerals. The reason for lumping them in one chapter is that we do not need to consume separate foods for each vitamin or mineral. A liberal intake of green vegetables, fruits and whole grains ensures an adequate supply of most of the vitamins and minerals. Therefore, we either get enough of all vitamins and minerals, or we get multiple deficiencies. Of course, there are exceptions to this general rule, and that is why we need to discuss this further.

Vitamins

Vitamin A is necessary for normal vision. Its deficiency, when mild, makes it difficult to see clearly in the dark; and when severe, may lead to blindness. Getting enough of vitamin A is not difficult. It is found in yellow and red fruits and vegetables, particularly in carrots, and to some extent, also in green leafy vegetables. Moreover, if the diet has a surplus of vitamin A, it can be stored in the liver. Therefore, having plenty of carrots in winters can see us through the summers as well.

Vitamin B is a family of vitamins, collectively called the B complex. Green vegetables, particularly leafy ones, and whole grains, can give us enough of B complex to meet our needs. Folic acid (or Folate) is a member of the B complex family, and its deficiency can have particularly serious consequences during pregnancy. Therefore, it is customary to supplement the diet with folic acid tablets during pregnancy. Vitamin B_{12} is unique in being a vitamin that is present only in animal foods. Therefore, vegetarians depend on milk and milk products for this vitamin. That is why vegan diets, which advocate not consuming any animal products whatsoever, and fruitarian diets, which are even more restricted, are likely to be deficient in vitamin B_{12} and a few other nutrients. A composite look at five studies published in 1999 in the *American Journal of Clinical Nutrition* indicated that although vegan as well as vegetarian diets reduce the risk of death due to coronary heart disease as compared to non-vegetarian diets, the protection offered by a lacto-ovo-vegetarian diet (diet having milk and egg but otherwise vegetarian) is slightly better than that by a vegan diet.

Vitamin C deficiency may lead to bleeding from the gums, or even full-blown scurvy. Indian gooseberry (amla) and fresh citrus fruits, such as oranges and lemons, are well-known as good sources of vitamin C. But most people are surprised to know that peas and papaya are among the richest sources of vitamin C. Fresh green leafy vegetables in general, if taken regularly in a decent amount, can also give us the required amount of this vitamin.

Vitamin D, often called the 'sunshine vitamin', is manufactured in the body when the skin is exposed to sunlight. However, living in a place with plenty of sunshine does not guarantee an adequate supply of vitamin D. Very few of us spend enough time in the sun with enough skin exposed to fully reap the benefits of this source. Therefore, drinking milk is important to get enough of vitamin D. Vitamin D helps in the absorption of calcium. Since milk has plenty of calcium, drinking milk is a good way of getting enough calcium as well as absorbing it properly.

After going through several phases of controversy, it seems quite certain now that we do need some vitamin E too, although not in the large doses found in some supplements. Vitamin E requirement depends partly on the type of fat we consume; the requirement is more if the dietary fat is unsaturated. Nature has, however, taken care of this factor—the more unsaturated an oil is, the higher is its vitamin E content.

Vitamin K is one of the substances that the body needs to stop bleeding from an injury. Vitamin K helps the blood clot at the site of injury. Green vegetables can take care of vitamin K intake.

Minerals

Iron is the one mineral that is commonly deficient in our diet. Its deficiency leads to anaemia, or inadequate haemoglobin in the blood. Anaemia leads to inadequate stamina, and a tendency to quickly get tired and breathless*. Anaemia is more common in women because their iron requirement is higher than that of men. This is so because women lose blood during menstruation, and also need additional iron during pregnancy and lactation. However, a balanced diet with adequate amounts of green vegetables, fruits and whole grains can look after iron needs. Non-vegetarians can also get iron from flesh foods, particularly liver. But it is customary, and safer, to take an iron supplement during the latter part of pregnancy and during lactation[†].

---

*But everyone who gets easily tired or breathless does not necessarily have anaemia.
[†]Taking an iron supplement during early pregnancy might do some harm. Therefore, pregnant women should take iron supplements during pregnancy only on a doctor's advice. In general, during pregnancy, any medicinal product (even a tablet for pain or fever) should be taken only after consulting a doctor.

Calcium is the other mineral that may be deficient in the diet. It is required for healthy bones and teeth. As mentioned earlier, it should be accompanied by vitamin D for the calcium to be absorbed properly. Both calcium and vitamin D may be obtained from milk and milk products. Most calcium supplements contain vitamin D as well. These supplements are commonly prescribed during pregnancy and lactation.

Iodine is yet another mineral that is deficient in the diet in some regions of the world. In India, iodine deficiency was very common in the sub-Himalayan belt, but it has been controlled quite effectively with the use of iodized salt. Mild forms of iodine deficiency also occur in coastal areas and in the plains. Therefore, it is desirable to consume iodized salt, irrespective of where a person lives. Iodine deficiency impairs thyroid function, and affects the development of a baby's brain even before it is born. As a result, the child is born with sub-normal mental function, which cannot be corrected by giving iodine later in life*.

How much fruit and vegetables should one have?

As is clear from the above discussion, having plenty of fruits and vegetables, particularly green leafy vegetables,

---

*Not all cases of impairment of thyroid function in adult life are due to iodine deficiency. Therefore, thyroxin tablets, rather than iodine, might be required for treatment of hypothyroidism (inadequate thyroid function) in adults.

is the simplest way of meeting our requirement of most of the vitamins and minerals. 'Plenty' here means about 500 grams (half a kilo) of fruits and vegetables put together. A convenient way to take that quantity is to have five to six helpings of these foods everyday. As a moderate helping is about 100 grams, five helpings give the required amount. One may eat a fruit at breakfast, some salad and a cooked vegetable at lunch, a fruit in the evening and some salad and a cooked vegetable at dinner. That makes six helpings of fruits and vegetables. Fruits and vegetables comprise one category of food that is taken in amounts far less than desirable even by those who can afford it. This happens due to a variety of reasons. One, fruits and vegetables are not considered very palatable by many*. Two, they take time and effort to chew, not to speak of the time required for peeling, cutting and cooking. Three, there is a general feeling that the vegetable (or dal) is required only to make the chapatti or rice more palatable. Therefore, the minimum amount that will achieve this end is considered enough. It is important to realize that fruits and vegetables deserve an independent place in the diet on their own merit. Fruits and vegetables supply us nutrients which no other food can in adequate amounts.

---

*It is all in the mind. There is really no good reason why the sweetness of a carrot, an apple or a pear should be considered less palatable than that of a barfi, a rasgulla or chocolate.

To supplement or not to supplement?

The standard answer to this difficult question has been that if the diet is healthy and balanced, supplementation is unnecessary. However, since it is difficult to be sure about how satisfactory one's diet is, and slight excess in intake of most of the vitamins is harmless, there is no harm in taking a vitamin–mineral supplement. While supplements continue to be used extensively, recent work has cast some doubts on their safety and efficacy. On the one hand, the number of vitamins that might prove to be harmful if taken in excess has increased. On the other hand, there is some evidence that vitamins contained in a pill may not be as effective as in natural foods. Therefore, vitamin–mineral pills might fail to provide the sort of insurance against deficiency for which they are commonly consumed. Thus, the pendulum is swinging away from pills towards natural foods. But there is probably still some justification for taking supplements during periods of excessive requirement. The requirement for some vitamins and minerals goes up during illnesses, especially when a person is on antibiotics, during pregnancy and lactation, and during stressful periods, such as after surgery. One simple precaution that might provide their benefit, if any, without the potential harm, is to take the supplements in moderation. One should never consume supplements that contain mega-doses of any vitamin or mineral.

Frequently Asked Questions

Are fruits and vegetables exchangeable?

The chemical composition of fruits and vegetables is similar. Most of them have more than 80 per cent water, very little energy-giving nutrients and at least some vitamins and minerals in good quantities. The main difference between the two is that fruits are generally eaten uncooked, while vegetables are cooked. Cooking leads to leaching of some of the vitamins and minerals in water that may be thrown away, and also to loss of some heat-labile vitamins. However, there are several vegetables that may also be had uncooked. Such vegetables become equivalent to fruits. Keeping practical considerations in mind, one may consume some fruit, some uncooked vegetables and some cooked vegetables too, the total number of servings per day being five or six.

Which is better—fruit or fruit juice?

Fruit includes the fruit juice, and is therefore better. Besides juice, the whole fruit also has at least some fibre that is thrown away when the juice is extracted. There is also one more important consideration that makes the whole fruit better. It is very easy to consume, for example, the juice of four oranges. But it is quite difficult to consume four oranges at one sitting. The result is that with fruit juice we are likely to consume more energy and more sugar, which is generally not desirable.

What is osteoporosis?

Osteoporosis is wasting and weakening of the bones. To an extent, it is inevitable with age, but the problem arises when bone loss is so marked that even a minor fall might lead to a fracture. The major risk factors for dangerous levels of osteoporosis are: inadequate calcium in the diet, lack of exercise and smoking. In women, there are some additional risk factors: not taking enough calcium during periods of heavy demand—such as pregnancy and lactation—and menopause.

There are a few important things to bear in mind in relation to osteoporosis. First, calcium deposition in bones takes place only during childhood and youth. Later on, it is only the loss that can be slowed down. In other words, it is not possible to reverse the bone loss in old age. Therefore, the right thing to do is to be conscious of this problem while still young, and build up a good bone density. If we start with a good stock, the depletion in old age can be tolerated better. Second, the diet may contain enough calcium, but that is of no use unless it is absorbed from the intestines. For absorbing calcium, vitamin D is important. Third, while the importance of calcium is widely appreciated, not enough attention is paid to physical exercise. Fourth, for prevention of osteoporosis, weight-bearing exercises are much more useful than simple stretches. Fifth, smoking is injurious to health for many reasons—to all those reasons one may add enhanced risk of osteoporosis. Sixth, even with a balanced diet, calcium supplements may be necessary during pregnancy and lactation. Finally, the risk of osteoporosis does not necessarily justify hormone replacement therapy (HRT)* during menopause. On the whole, informed medical opinion is currently not in favour of long-term HRT. It may be relevant to add here that Bone Mineral Density (BMD) as a predictor of osteoporotic fractures is itself under a scanner—therefore, it may not be prudent to go in for aggressive therapy simply because the BMD is marginally below some arbitrary standards.

SUMMARY

1. Although required in small amounts, vitamins and several minerals are essential nutrients.
2. A liberal intake of green vegetables, fruits and whole grains ensures an adequate supply of most of the vitamins and minerals.
3. A healthy diet has at least five moderate helpings of fruits and vegetables everyday.

---

*Hormone Replacement Therapy (HRT) is sometimes given to women to treat menopausal symptoms. HRT consists of the female hormone, estrogen, with or without the other female hormone, progesterone. While short-term HRT (less than one year) is not harmful, the effects of long-term HRT (more than five years) are mixed. While it does seem to reduce the risk of osteoporosis, it may increase the risk of coronary heart disease and stroke.

6
The Universal Friend

Varuna represents largeness, right and purity; everything that deviates from the right, from the purity, recoils from his being and strikes the offender as the punishment of sin.

SRI AUROBINDO,
on Varuna (the god of water),
in *The Secret of the Veda*

Water is a nutrient, but is generally taken for granted. However, the fact is that life originated in water, and even within the animals that live on land (human beings included), each cell of the body has a tiny little private pond, to nourish it and to accept its waste. One can live without food much longer than without water.

How much water do we need?

We need just enough water to balance the losses. The losses are primarily through urine and sweat. The amount of water lost in sweat depends on the weather. In summers, the loss is further enhanced if we are outdoors and exert physically. In short, the water requirement of an adult may vary from about 1 to 5 litres a day. Fortunately, we do not have to worry much about how much water we need on a particular day. There are two guides to tell us how much water to drink—thirst and the colour of urine. If we depend only on thirst, we may get just enough water, but just enough is not good enough; a little more is better. The colour of urine can guide us towards that. If we drink enough water to ensure that urine is essentially colourless rather than yellow, that water intake is more than 'just enough', and that is desirable.

Why should we drink a little more water than is essential?

Drinking a little more water than is strictly necessary is in the interest of our kidneys. The kidneys are so designed that if we drink less water, they concentrate the urine, with the result that the urine colour is deep yellow. On the other hand, if we drink more water, the same waste products are thrown out by the kidneys in a larger volume of water. The result is dilute, colourless urine. Dilute urine is safe urine. Dilute urine prevents two of the most common diseases of the kidneys: kidney stones and infections. Stones start as tiny crystals, but this crystallization is less likely if the urine has more water and less of the solids dissolved in it. Therefore, if the urine stays dilute, the risk of getting urinary stones goes down. Germs also need food material to grow on, and therefore, grow more easily in concentrated urine. Dilute urine, which is essentially all water, cannot support the growth of germs. Therefore, urinary tract infections are also less likely if the urine is dilute. Sips of water are what it takes, to keep the kidneys in good shape!

Closing thoughts

Water is cheap and abundant, but seldom clean. Clean, potable water is a luxury in India. If the water is unfit for drinking, it is possible to make it drinkable by boiling it. Bottled water, which has not only been disinfected but also treated to achieve a specific electrolyte composition, is generally safe in the short term. But its long-term use is questionable for several reasons. One, it is not certain whether bottled water is truly safer than chlorinated tap water. Two, the long-term health effects of the doctored electrolyte composition of bottled water are controversial. Three, storage in plastic bottles introduces certain chemicals into the water, the safety of which is uncertain. Finally, large-scale consumption of bottled water contributes significantly to environmental depletion and pollution. In short, for a large population, chlorination; and for families, boiling continue to be the least expensive and least controversial options for making drinking water safe.

Frequently Asked Questions

What is the best time to have water in relation to a meal?

There are many advocates of drinking no water with a meal, as well as of drinking water before, during or after a meal. Each of these options has a rationale.

- Water dilutes the digestive juices. Therefore, drinking water with meals weakens digestion. Hence, one should not drink water at mealtime.
- Drinking water before a meal fills up the tummy. Therefore, it helps in eating less. Hence, one should have water just before a meal if one wants to lose weight.
- Having water during the meal helps in rinsing the mouth between morsels. Therefore, drinking water a few times during the meal helps in enjoying the unmixed taste of each item.
- Consuming water after a meal serves as a partial mouthwash. Therefore, it helps in keeping the teeth healthy.

What is the last word then? Well, not exactly the last word, but my considered opinion is that:

(a) one may have water before a meal, and
(b) even more important, the water taken with a meal should not be more than one glass.

The rationale for this advice is that up to one glass of water does not dilute the digestive juices much, and is therefore compatible with good digestion. Having this one glass will help achieve a good water intake, because many people remember to have water only at mealtimes. Drinking water before meals is not just for losing weight; overeating is not good for us, irrespective of our body weight. There is a dictum in Ayurveda that at mealtimes, one should imagine the capacity of the stomach, and then fill one quarter with water, two quarters with food and leave the remaining quarter empty! In other words, one does not have to go on eating till it is impossible to eat any more. The rinsing of the mouth during the meal to enjoy the unmixed taste is something that does not seem important to me. Washing one's mouth after the meal is important, but one might as well have a thorough mouth wash after the meal instead of depending on the partial mouth wash achieved by drinking water*.

How can one have water in the evening, and avoid getting disturbed during sleep?

This question is particularly important for elderly men who have an enlarged prostate, and therefore have a tendency to get up at night to pass urine. If they drink a lot of water close to their bedtime, they have to get up even more often. This dilemma may be solved by

---

*One might, however, use drinking water (or tea without sugar and milk) to wash the mouth if it is difficult to go for a thorough mouth wash (for example, if a bathroom is not accessible). Even a partial mouth wash is better than not washing the mouth at all.

their having an early dinner (at least two hours before bedtime), having water with dinner but not after that, and passing urine just before going to bed. The natural question that arises is whether that will make the urine concentrated, and therefore, unsafe. There is a bit of compromise involved here, but one may correct this problem by drinking plenty of water (at least two glasses) soon after getting up in the morning. This water would flush the kidneys, and undo the adverse effects, if any, of the somewhat concentrated urine formed overnight. From this point of view, drinking plenty of water early in the morning is good for everyone.

Is water alone enough to replace sweat losses?

Sweat has water as well as electrolytes. Therefore, if the sweat losses are heavy, it is better to have water with some lemon and a pinch of salt added to it.

Is it possible to drink too much water?

Yes, there can be too much of a good thing. One, there are people who sometimes develop a neurotic tendency to drink water again and again. That is inconvenient, and may be harmful. And two, there are some diseases in which doctors restrict water intake, salt intake, or both. In such cases, it is best to follow the doctor's advice.

How does water compare with carbonated drinks?

Carbonated drinks (aerated drinks or sodas) damage the teeth. This choice has to be made frequently while travelling, when the option may be between sodas and bottled water. Of the two, bottled water is the healthier option. Tea, especially without sugar, is also a good option because it contains boiled water.

SUMMARY

1. The amount of water we drink should be a little more than is strictly necessary.
2. There are two guides to tell us how much water to drink— thirst and the colour of urine. Of course, one should respond to thirst, but it is better to take more water than is strictly necessary to satisfy thirst. One should also try to ensure that the urine is colourless rather than deep yellow.
3. Dilute urine prevents two of the most common diseases of the kidneys: stones and infections.
4. At mealtimes, water should be limited to less than one glass, which is best taken at the beginning of the meal.

7
New Kids on the Block

A circuit ending where it first began
Is dubbed the forward and eternal march
Of progress on perfection's unknown road.

Sri Aurobindo
Savitri, Book 2, Canto 6

Carbohydrates, proteins, fats, vitamins, minerals and water are the six broad categories of chemicals that have traditionally been considered nutrients. But food also has small quantities of several chemicals that do not fall under any of these six categories. For a long time, these additional substances were considered passive and redundant components of food. However, research during the last few decades has thrown new light on them. It is being increasingly realized that the functions of food need not be restricted to providing energy and building the body for growth and repair. The functions may be extended to include strengthening our immunity and other protective mechanisms of the body. Thus, prevention of disease is also one of the functions of food, and this may be due to chemicals other than the traditional nutrients. Foods, which are rich in these protective chemicals, have been somewhat erroneously called 'functional foods' to signify the fact that their functions go beyond those of traditional nutrients. Thus, curd (yogurt), which has 'friendly' germs that improve local immunity of the intestines and thereby prevent diarrhoea, is a functional food. Similarly, tomato, which contains the anti-cancer chemical, lycopene, is also a functional food. Spices, earlier thought to contribute only to the taste and fragrance of the food, also have several protective factors, and are therefore functional foods.

Unlike in the case of traditional nutrients, identifying the new non-traditional nutrients and assigning a specific function to each has not been easy. By now, hundreds of non-traditional nutrients have been detected, they have tongue-twisting chemical names and overlapping functions. One big group among these chemicals has antioxidant activity.

Antioxidants

Getting energy from food involves a process similar to burning wood. Wood burns with the help of oxygen in the air, and releases heat energy. Similarly, food burns with the help of the oxygen that we breathe, and releases energy that we use for staying alive and active.

The process involved in the release of energy is called oxidation. Thus, oxidation is essential for life. However, oxidation has an unpleasant by-product—it releases highly reactive chemical entities (called free radicals, or reactive oxygen species) that can cause serious damage to the cells of the body. To prevent this damage, we need antioxidants. There are two types of antioxidant mechanisms in the body. One is in-built; the other is dependant on certain dietary factors. The dietary factors with antioxidant activity belong to both the traditional and non-traditional nutrients. Among the traditional nutrients, vitamins A, C and E, and selenium (a mineral) have antioxidant activity. A few examples of non-traditional nutrients having antioxidant activity are: resveratrol and flavonoids in grapes and tea; lycopene in tomatoes, guavas and watermelons; lutein in spinach, carrots, corn, green vegetables and yellow fruits; and allyl sulphides in onion and garlic.

Why do we need antioxidants?

As mentioned earlier, antioxidants prevent cellular damage in the body. This translates into slower aging, better immunity against infections and reduced risk of cancer. It is quite possible that several of the other benefits of non-traditional nutrients are also the result of their antioxidant activity.

Other benefits of non-traditional nutrients

Besides antioxidant activity, the other beneficial effects that have been attributed to non-traditional nutrients are reduction in blood sugar and reduction in cholesterol levels. These effects translate into reduced risk of diabetes and heart disease.

How can we ensure adequate intake of non-traditional nutrients?

In spite of the complexities touched upon above, it is fortunately quite easy to get enough of the non-traditional nutrients from a regular diet. In order to see how, let us look at two basic facts. One, all the protective factors identified so far have been found in plant foods. For that reason, they are sometimes also called phytochemicals (phyto meaning plants). Two, although the number of individual protective factors runs into hundreds, their functions overlap, and therefore it is not essential to get each one of them everyday. Putting these two facts together, all that we need to do is to consume plenty of plant foods, especially fruits and vegetables, and to have a variety of them. In addition, we should also consume spices in moderation. Spices are a concentrated source of protective non-traditional nutrients. The spices that have been studied in some detail and shown to have beneficial effects are turmeric (haldi), ginger (adrak), and fenugreek (methi). In the meantime, we can continue taking other spices too—the beneficial effects of some of them (such as reduction of flatulence) are household knowledge in India, and have also been documented in Ayurveda. It would not be prudent to give up any of the traditional spices just because research has not yet rediscovered their beneficial effects.

Health foods and food supplements

The new knowledge summarized above has been exploited commercially in at least four ways.

One, some companies highlight the research on beneficial effects of certain foods, thereby pushing up their demand as well as the price. A case in point is walnut. Owing to the research indicating its tendency to protect against heart disease, the humble walnut is today among the most prestigious and expensive of nuts.

Two, they modify or fortify a normal food and present it as a health food. The health food is then sold at a much higher price than the normal food. For example, curd is fortified with active bacteria and sometimes also starchy material that promotes the growth of these bacteria. When we buy such expensive curd, we forget that the traditional curd–rice or parantha–curd combination, which uses homemade curd, is the same thing at a much lower cost. Or, ordinary biscuits may be modified by adding the calcium-rich grain, ragi. The question one should ask is, how much ragi does each biscuit contain? How much calcium will one biscuit give? How many biscuits would be required to meet even 25 per cent of the daily calcium requirement? Will that be cheaper and nutritionally more sound than getting the same amount of calcium from milk or milk products? The answers to such questions invariably are that one biscuit would supply a miniscule amount of calcium, and that to get a respectable amount of calcium, one would have to eat so many biscuits that it would be very expensive as well as lead to overeating. But the fact that the biscuits contain ragi, which is rich in calcium, is highlighted, and provides the apparent justification for the exorbitant price of the biscuits.

Three, they extract the 'active principle' from a food and pack it in a capsule or a pill. This is worse than the previous two strategies. For example, lycopene has been extracted from tomatoes and packed in capsules. The justification given is that the amount of the protective chemical in one pill comes from several kilos of the natural food. Since it is difficult to eat such a large quantity of the natural food, it is better to have the pill. The point that this argument misses is that we do not need such a large amount of any single protective factor. Small bits of different protective factors with similar functions from different foods would together give us the required protection. Not only that, there is now some evidence indicating that first, protective factors packed in pills may not be as effective as those in natural foods; and second, heroic doses of even the 'protective' factors may be harmful—there can be too much of a good thing.

Finally, the industry itself sponsors research on the foods they wish to promote. For example, the tea industry has sponsored research on tea. Such research shows that tea protects against heart disease, and the benefit is attributed to antioxidants. Then the industry goes about advertising the results of the research that they have sponsored. Even if we assume that these advertisements tell the truth, it is only part of the truth. What they hide are two important facts. One, they say nothing about the harmful effects of drinking large quantities of tea. Two, they do not inform us that tea is only one of the several foods containing antioxidants, and therefore it is possible to get all the antioxidants one needs even without having any tea at all. Similar research has also been sponsored by the coffee and chocolate industries. The results and claims are similar, and we need the same critical attitude while looking at news items based on such research.

Apart from looking at the advertisements and claims of health foods and supplements critically, it is important to remember that only the knowledge about non-traditional nutrients is new. Human beings have always needed these nutrients, and have been getting them from healthy and balanced diets without making any special effort. We might not have known the chemical names of all these nutrients, but we have been ingesting them in natural foods and have stayed healthy because of them.

Frequently Asked Questions

What are genetically modified foods?

No two human beings are alike because their genes are never the same. The variation is introduced by sexual reproduction, as a result of which each individual gets half of his or her genes from the father and half from the mother. Similar variation is seen in several plants as well. Further, the variation can be given a direction by the farmer, by bringing together the genes of two different plants of the same species, each of which has some desirable characteristics. By doing so, he may succeed in getting the desirable characteristics of both the plants in a single plant. Scientists helped farmers do so in the 1970s in a more efficient goal-directed manner, and that engineered the Green Revolution in India. But plants produced in this manner *are not* genetically modified (GM) plants. In GM plants, a gene is introduced into a plant from another species. For example, strawberries have been modified to withstand extremely cold climates by introducing the gene for an anti-freeze protein from a fish into the strawberry genes.

Are GM foods safe?

The simple answer is: nobody knows yet. Those who argue that they are safe say that GM foods have been consumed in the US for more than ten years without any apparent harm. They attribute the fears about safety to the natural tendency to resist change. Those who are against GM foods prefer to be cautious about trying foods produced by a fundamentally unprecedented process. It is impossible to say confidently that even slow and subtle harmful effects cannot arise from long-term consumption of large quantities of a large variety of GM foods. It has been pointed out, for example, that plants belonging to family Solanaceae frequently contain substances toxic to human beings. One of the members of Solanaceae is brinjal. Brinjal has been made toxin-free through 'natural' methods over hundreds of years. It is quite possible that the toxin might reappear in the GM brinjal. The argument is logical, but based on a very slender foundation. At the same time, it is impossible to dismiss the argument without a thorough study of the GM brinjal.

Are there any other concerns about GM foods?

More significant than the objections to GM foods based on potential health risks are those based on the social implications of GM foods. GM foods are the result of research sponsored by wealthy multinational companies (MNCs). These companies acquire patents for these foods, and control the sale of the seeds for these plants. The GM foods often produce seeds programmed to self-destruct. Hence, their seeds cannot be utilized by farmers. Fresh seeds have to be purchased year after year from the MNCs at the price dictated by them. Thus, GM foods have the potential to push the small farmer out of business, and hand over food production to giant MNCs. It does not seem prudent to be at the mercy of a few powerful companies for something as essential as food.

SUMMARY

1. Besides the six traditional nutrients—carbohydrates, proteins, fats, vitamins, minerals and water—there seem to be many other components of foods, present only in minute amounts, which have important functions that go beyond those of the traditional nutrients.
2. The number of non-traditional nutrients identified so far runs into hundreds, and they have overlapping functions. The functions assigned to them cover a wide range:

improving immune function; preventing heart disease, diabetes and cancer; and slowing down aging.

3. Many of the beneficial effects of non-traditional nutrients may be due to their antioxidant activity.

4. In order to ensure adequate intake of these nutrients, we should have plenty of fruits and vegetables, and also a variety of spices in moderation. In general, it is better to get our supply of these nutrients from natural foods, rather than health foods or nutritional supplements.

8

The Nitty-Gritty

Fad diets are bad diets.

What we need are nutrients, whereas what we eat are a variety of foods, each of which has one or more nutrients. For example, grains provide us mainly carbohydrates and proteins, while vegetables provide us mainly vitamins and minerals. Let us see how we can put the knowledge of our nutrient requirement and food composition together to frame a satisfactory diet.

We need food more for energy than for anything else. In the Indian diet, much of the energy comes from a mixture of cereals and pulses. This is an excellent combination because along with providing us carbohydrates for energy, it also gives us all the protein we need. Further, although cereal protein and pulse protein are individually of poor quality, together they make a good quality protein. Grains (cereals and pulses) do not contain much fat, but the small quantity that they do is of the type that is essential for us. In the absence of any other source of fat, the fat that we get from grains can take care of the minimum quantity of the fat that we need. If we consume the grains in an unrefined form, besides giving us carbohydrates, proteins and fats, they also give us dietary fibre. That is not all. Grains, especially in unrefined form, also make a significant contribution to our vitamin and mineral intake, but their contribution is not enough to meet our total requirement. In short, if our staple food consists of grains, we need other foods mainly to make up for the shortfall in vitamins and minerals.

The best sources of vitamins and minerals are fruits and vegetables. This is an oft-neglected part of the Indian diet. We need five helpings of fruits and vegetables a day to meet our requirements. This is easily accomplished by eating a fruit at breakfast, and a cooked vegetable and a salad at lunch as well as dinner. Fruit (usually consumed uncooked) and uncooked vegetables (in salads) are helpful because cooking generally leads to a reduction in the vitamin and mineral content of the food. Apart from providing us vitamins and minerals, fruits and vegetables also give us dietary fibre. The fibre that we get from fruits and vegetables is chemically somewhat different from that which we get from cereals. The fibres from these two sources also differ in their metabolic effects. Therefore, it is important to get some fibre from each of these sources.

Are there any vitamins and minerals that we may still not get enough of, even if we consume grains as well as fruits and vegetables? Yes, we may still not get enough of calcium, and vitamin B_{12}. For both these very important nutrients, vegetarians depend on milk and milk products. Curd is better than milk because it is easier to digest, and also has a higher content of certain vitamins. Curd may also improve local immunity of the gut, thereby preventing diarrhoea.

A diet that has cereals, pulses, vegetables, fruits, milk and milk products may be enough to prevent any obvious nutritional deficiency, but may still not be optimal for good health and prevention of disease. For these additional legitimate expectations from food, an adequate supply of non-traditional nutrients is also important. That is where spices come to our rescue. Spices are a concentrated source of non-traditional nutrients, as well as several vitamins and minerals.

Although a diet that has cereals, pulses, vegetables, fruits, milk and milk products, and spices may be completely satisfactory, it may not be palatable or practical unless we also include some fats and oils, sugar, and salt. These are all industrial products. Before these products became available, man survived for centuries without them. However, the human body is resilient enough to tolerate these products in moderation without any significant harm. The key word is moderation in quantity. Further, in relation to fats, besides moderation in quantity, the type of fat consumed also has some bearing on chronic disease.

A diet, which is satisfactory from the scientific point of view, is generally called a balanced diet. A balanced diet is a vegetarian diet (or at least predominantly so), which contains:

(a) A mixture of cereals and pulses, consumed whole (unrefined) as far as possible, as the staple food.
(b) Five helpings a day of fruits and vegetables, especially the green leafy vegetables.
(c) Milk or milk products in moderation.
(d) Spices in moderation.
(e) Moderate quantity of judiciously chosen fats.
(f) Sugar and salt in moderation.

As is obvious, the diet given above is a simple diet, without any exotic foods. Therefore, to eat a healthy and balanced diet is easy. It is especially easy for Indians because this diet is essentially a good Indian diet. It may be a hardship for people accustomed to European, Russian or North American diets because over the last hundred years or so, the wealthy nations of the world have got accustomed to high-fat, high-sugar diets in which the staple food is meat. Such diets are palatable, but there is enough scientific evidence to show that they are extremely unhealthy. It is very easy to become overweight on these diets. Being low in fibre, these diets promote constipation and all its sequelae, such as piles and varicose veins. Being high in energy and fat content these diets increase the risk of diabetes and heart disease. Excess of fat, lack of fibre and eating meat have also been linked to several cancers. Hence the world is turning to whole grains, fruits and vegetables, and is cutting down on fats, sugar, salt and meat. The rationale for a balanced diet has been summarized in Table 8.1.

Table 8.1. The constituents and rational basis of a balanced diet

Food	What we need it for the most
Cereals and pulses*	Energy and proteins, dietary fibre
Fruits and vegetables	Dietary fibre, vitamins and minerals, non-traditional nutrients
Spices	Vitamins and minerals, non-traditional nutrients
Milk and milk products	Calcium, vitamin B_{12}
Fats and oils	Not essential, but acceptable in moderation
Sugar	Not essential, but acceptable in moderation
Salt	Not essential, but acceptable in moderation

How much?

We have talked so far about what a balanced diet should have. Besides what we eat, the effect food has on health depends on how much we eat. To some extent, a healthy diet makes it easier to also eat the right quantity of food. A healthy diet is a high-fibre diet, which is neither very palatable nor easy to eat. Such a diet contains foods that have to be chewed properly before they can be swallowed. Therefore, it takes effort and time to eat a healthy meal. Studies have shown that, irrespective of the energy content of a meal, a person feels satiated after he has spent about twenty minutes on eating. Therefore, if the meals are healthy, it is almost impossible to overeat. Besides the in-built mechanisms of hunger and satiation, the other guide to how much we should eat is the body

---

*If consumed unrefined (i.e. with the husk intact).

weight. If the body weight is stable, it means that the food intake and requirements are fairly well-matched*.

Losing weight

Obesity is a major public health problem in urban India today. With about a quarter of the population, including children, weighing more than they should, we are catching up fast with many countries in the West. Excessive weight is due to energy imbalance, which can be the result of eating too much, exercising too little or both. This basic fact remains true even when it is the 'hormones' or 'genes' that add to the risk. Preventing and treating obesity is important because it is the mother of many maladies; a partial list includes high blood pressure, heart disease, diabetes, gallstones, menstrual problems, some cancers, osteoarthritis and sleep apnoea. Losing weight is one area in which whatever is good is not new; and whatever is new is not good. The best treatment

---

*'Fairly well-matched', but not exactly so, because the body can adapt, to some extent, to both a deficient intake and an excessive intake without this being visible through body weight. Neither of these situations is desirable. Adaptation to deficient intake may be accompanied by impaired immunity, thereby making the person vulnerable to repeated bouts of common cold or diarrhoea. Adaptation to excessive intake may be accompanied by a higher risk for high blood pressure, heart disease or diabetes. Hence, moderation is the golden rule, and it is easy to stick to the golden rule if the diet is balanced and healthy.

has two time-honoured components: eating less and exercising more. Newer approaches, such as drugs and surgery, should be only the last resort.

Diet

An adult trying to lose weight should follow a 1,000–1,500 Calorie diet. A dietician can help convert this figure into dietary recommendations requiring minimum change in dietary habits. In general, everything that a person consumes should be reduced in quantity, with greater emphasis on sweets and high-fat foods. To ensure that the person does not remain hungry in spite of reducing the energy intake, the quantity of fruits and uncooked vegetables should be increased. Further, the person should cultivate the habits of eating slowly and chewing the food well.

The sequence in which a person eats can also help. The best items to start with are water, salads and sweets, and there is a rationale for each. A glass of water taken at the beginning of the meal makes a person feel full, and therefore he is unlikely to overeat. Salad has very little energy content, but is filling. Therefore, if the beginning is made with salad, again, the person is unlikely to overeat. If a sweet (dessert) is also a part of the meal, it is best taken in the beginning because it will raise the blood sugar fast, and thereby wipe away hunger. Therefore, after eating the sweet, the person will compensate for its energy content by eating less of the other foods in the meal. In contrast, if the sweet is taken at the end of the meal, it is generally in addition to what the person needs.

Even after a person reaches a point where he cannot have more rice or chapattis, he still welcomes an ice cream.

It is not advisable to go in for crash diets, fad diets or total exclusion of 'fattening foods'. In fact, there are no fattening or slimming foods. If the energy intake exceeds the expenditure, any diet, no matter what it includes or what it excludes, will lead to weight gain. Therefore, it is desirable to reduce energy intake by making modest changes in the dietary pattern to which a person is accustomed. Drastic changes in the diet are unlikely to last and may also be detrimental. To make the dietary changes more effective, they should be accompanied by an increase in the energy expenditure.

Exercise

Exercise may be a part of everyday activities, or a special slot may be created for it. Both are desirable, for those who want to lose weight as well as for others. In the course of everyday activities, it is healthy to make use of every opportunity for physical activity—for example, by choosing to walk instead of taking a vehicle and by choosing to climb the stairs instead of taking the lift or the escalator. In addition, a slot for regular, structured exercise is also part of a healthy lifestyle. The simplest exercise is a thirty-minute brisk walk. One may walk longer, do yogic postures and breathing practices, go to the gym or whatever a person likes and finds suitable. Sedentary persons starting exercise after a long time, those above forty and those having high blood pressure or heart disease or some other chronic illness, should consult their doctor before starting on an exercise programme.

Gaining weight

Although there are not many who want to gain weight, some people are not very happy about the fact that they do not put on weight, no matter how much they eat. If they are otherwise healthy, they just need reassurance. They should eat well, but stick to a healthy diet. They should also remain physically active, which may appear unnecessary for them, but helps in at least three ways. First, exercise improves general health and the level of fitness. Second, exercise improves appetite, which is useful for those who wish to gain weight. Finally, exercise increases muscle mass; it is much better to put on muscles than fat.

Closing thoughts

Besides what we eat and how much we eat, the attitude with which we eat also determines how food affects us. This important aspect of eating will be discussed in Chapter 10.

Frequently Asked Questions

What are the functions of foods?

The time-honoured functions of food are just two: to provide energy and to build the body. We need some amount of energy just to stay alive (e.g. for the pumping action of the heart, and for breathing). We need some more energy for physical activity. We also need a little bit of energy to digest and utilize food. We need to build the body so that the cells lost through wear and tear can be replaced. In addition, children need to build the body for growth. Some nutrients do not contribute directly to these two functions, but are still essential.

Besides the two time-honoured functions of food, now, it has been discovered that food can also make a contribution towards maintenance of optimal health through its anti-oxidant, immuno-enhancing, anti-infective, hypolipidemic, hypoglycemic and anti-cancer effects. These 'non-traditional' functions of food have been discussed in Chapter 7.

What is The China Study?

The China Study was one of the most comprehensive dietary surveys ever conducted. It covered more than 2,400 Chinese counties, and its findings revealed more than 8,000 associations between dietary factors and disease. Based on the study, the leader of the team that conducted it, Professor Colin Campbell of Cornell University, and his son, Thomas, published a book of the same name in 2005. The book contains a lot more than the findings of the China Study. It is a well-researched and referenced book, and brings between its covers authentic wisdom on nutrition, which has behind it Dr Campbell's teaching experience of more than forty years, his research, committee work and strikingly honest introspection. It explodes many common myths about nutrition, and also explains why these abound, in spite of ample evidence against them. What is worse, it points out, is that the simple and sane principles of healthy nutrition get buried under a mountain of motivated propaganda. This happens because 'The entire system—government, science, medicine, industry and media—promotes profits over health, technology over food and confusion over clarity'.*

What is BMI?

BMI stands for Body Mass Index. It is a criterion for classifying people into 'normal weight' and 'overweight'. Mathematically, BMI = Weight (in kg) / [Height (in metres)]^2. For example, if a person weighs 60 kg, and his height is 165 cm (1.65 metres), then his BMI = 60 / [1.65 x 1.65] = 60 / 2.72 = 22. According to Western standards, if a person's BMI is between 19 and 25, he is considered 'normal' in weight. For Indians, the normal BMI is between 19 and 23. Anybody having a BMI below 19 is considered underweight, and runs the risk of lowered immunity. For Indians, BMI above 23 is an indicator of being overweight and is associated with hypertension, heart disease and diabetes.

What is yo-yo dieting?

Yo-yo dieting is a term used for losing and gaining weight repeatedly. It often results from adopting a drastic diet for losing weight. The diet is unpalatable, requires major

---

*Campbell, Colin T. and Thomas M. Campbell. *The China Study: Startling Implication for Diet, Weight Loss and Long-term Health*. Texas: Benbella Books, 2006 (p. 250)

changes in the person's dietary habits and leaves the person hungry. However, the person sticks to it for the sake of losing weight. He does lose weight rather fast, but pretty soon comes temptation and an excuse to succumb to it. Then he is back to the old accustomed food habits and gains all the lost weight back. The process may be repeated several times, resulting in a 'yo-yo' phenomenon, so called because the weight goes up and down, again and again, somewhat like the yo-yo that children play with.

Why is yo-yo dieting undesirable, and how can it be avoided?

Yo-yo dieting is considered undesirable because there is some evidence that it may be associated with reduction in lifespan and onset of diabetes. It has also been linked to many other risks, but the evidence is controversial. But there is general agreement that sustained weight loss is better than the yo-yo phenomenon. The yo-yo phenomenon can be prevented by following the path of moderation. The diet adopted for losing weight should be healthy, balanced, filling and not very different from the one to which the person is accustomed. Such a diet should be combined with moderate increase in physical activity. One should not expect a spectacular fall in body weight. Further, if there is an inherent tendency of being overweight, one might have to be satisfied with shedding only a part of the excess weight. Just as there is a range of normal heights, there is also a range of normal weights. Everybody cannot achieve size zero, and it is not necessary either.

Is fasting good for health?

Prolonged or too frequent fasting or starvation is certainly not good for health, even if undertaken for losing weight. If undertaken for losing weight, it is likely to lead to the yo-yo effect, which is undesirable. However, occasional fasting, such as missing a meal once a week, is good for at least three reasons—biological, philosophical and spiritual.

Biological

Getting three to four meals a day at regular intervals is a recent phenomenon in human history. Before that, people ate whenever food was available; and sometimes food was not available for long periods of time. Survival under conditions of food deprivation is ensured by several mechanisms, which mobilize the body's reserves. If we always have three to four meals in a day, we do not give these mechanisms a chance to work. If any ability of the body is not used, it is weakened by disuse. For example, if muscles are used in exercise, they grow stronger; if they are not used, the muscles become weak. Similarly, in order to keep our capacity to mobilize reserves strong, we should use it frequently by deliberately missing a meal or two.

Philosophical

Fasting develops self-control, which makes life easier and happier. If, on any day, it becomes difficult to get a meal (e.g. due to lack of time or the inability to find a satisfactory meal at an acceptable price), the person is undaunted and just says to himself, 'I can easily miss a meal. I know nothing will happen to me because I fast regularly anyway.'

<u>Spiritual</u>

Scarcity of food is a reality in the world even today. Millions of people in the world sleep hungry because they have no choice. A periodic fast, which gives us a glimpse of how these starving millions feel, can be a spiritually uplifting experience, if we think of them with compassion during the fast and do something to convert this empathy into action. For example, if I travel on a 'no-frills' airline, I have the choice of missing a meal or spending ₹100 on a sandwich. If I make a conscious choice to miss a meal, and instead spend the hundred rupees on feeding five hungry persons, I will hit three birds with one stone. One, I will jog my body's mechanisms for mobilizing reserves. Two, I will improve my self-control. Three, I will grow spiritually because I have not missed the meal to save money, but out of love for my fellow beings.

<u>Caution</u>

Those who are on medication for diabetes should not fast. If they miss a meal, medication, even if taken twelve hours earlier, might give them a dangerously low level of blood sugar (hypoglycemia).

What are the effects of caffeinated drinks on health?

Coffee, tea and colas are the major caffeinated liquids. They are not essential, but are consumed extensively and, in moderation, the caffeine that they provide is almost harmless. The quantity of caffeine that is considered completely safe is 100 mg of caffeine per day, an amount present in one cup of coffee or two cups of tea or two cola drinks.

Caffeine improves physical and mental performance if it has been impaired by exhaustion or lack of sleep. But caffeine might also make a person anxious, agitated, jittery or irritable. If taken close to bedtime, in some individuals, caffeine might interfere with sleep. Those having heartburn, acidity or peptic ulcer experience an aggravation of symptoms if they consume a caffeinated drink.

Caffeinated drinks may have health effects that are due to components other than caffeine. For example, research during the last few decades has shown that tea and coffee have a protective effect against heart disease and cancer. The protective effect has been attributed to the antioxidants in tea and coffee. What this research has found is true, but is only part of the truth. Antioxidants are found not only in tea and coffee, but also in fruits, vegetables, spices and other plant foods. Therefore, a person does not have to tolerate the ill effects of tea and coffee for the sake of antioxidants.

What are the effects of alcohol on health?

The acute effects of alcohol are due to what it does to the nervous system. Under the influence of alcohol, a person becomes uninhibited and talkative. His driving skills suffer because of errors in judgement, over-confidence and unsteady limbs.

The commonest and most predictable long-term effect of alcohol is liver disease: generally cirrhosis and sometimes, cancer of the liver. Liver disease is progressive, essentially incurable and eventually a fatal problem.

During the last few decades, a considerable amount of research has been conducted on the possibility of alcohol having a protective effect against heart disease. The results of the research have been conflicting. It is also possible that the protective effect, if any, is due to either reduction in mental stress or due to the antioxidants present in wine. Putting all the facts known so far together, there is no good case for recommending alcohol for its protective effect. Alcohol can hardly add to the protection offered by a prudent diet and exercise, but can certainly increase the risk of liver disease and several other health-related and social problems.

However, if a person must imbibe alcohol, the safe limit for men is one glass (200 ml) of wine, or two glasses of beer, or two pegs (60 ml, diluted to two glasses) of whisky. Women, due to biological reasons, are less tolerant to alcohol. Therefore, the safe limit for women is half that for men. During pregnancy and lactation, women are advised to avoid alcohol altogether.

The best option, however, is not to drink alcohol at all. Alcohol in any quantity poses additional risks for those having high blood pressure, irregular heartbeat (arrhythmias), liver disease, peptic ulcer, sleep apnoea or breast cancer. Those on any medication should also check with their doctor whether alcohol interacts with the drugs they are taking. Alcohol interacts dangerously with several commonly taken drugs such as painkillers, sleeping pills, tranquillizers, anti-depressants, blood thinners (anticoagulants) and antihistaminics.

What is the Atkins diet?

Based on his personal positive experience of losing weight on a low-carbohydrate diet, Dr Robert Atkins published a book, *Dr. Atkins' Diet Revolution,* in 1972. The book was revised, and renamed *Dr. Atkins' New Diet Revolution* in 2001, but the basic philosophy, of using a low carbohydrate diet for losing weight, remained intact. The theory behind the philosophy is that if the diet is low in carbohydrates, the body will be forced to use stored fat as fuel. Although apparently logical, the theory is rather flawed. First, the body will use stored fat while the person is on a low-carbohydrate diet only if the total energy content of the diet is less than the energy expenditure; otherwise, the person can use dietary fat and protein as fuel, and will still store surplus energy, if any, as fat. As Dr Atkins conceded, his diet is not a licence to gorge on high protein and high-fat foods. Second, the body uses stored fat as fuel even if the diet is high in carbohydrates, provided the energy content of the diet is less than the energy expenditure. Third, research on the safety of the Atkins diet has given conflicting results.

The Atkins diet has four phases. The first phase, the induction phase, allows only 20 g of carbohydrates per day, and has several other dos and don'ts associated with it. Depending upon how much weight a person has to lose, this phase may last several weeks. The next phase, the on-going weight loss phase, allows an increase in the intake of carbohydrates by 5 g/day every week. This phase lasts till the weight loss is within 4.5 kg (10 pounds) of the target weight. The third phase, the pre-maintenance phase, allows a further increase in the intake of carbohydrates by 10 g/day every week. The aim is to find the critical carbohydrate intake level permissible for weight maintenance. It is doubtful if this concept of the critical level has any sound physiological basis. The last phase, the lifetime maintenance phase, emphasizes the need for being careful about one's diet throughout one's life. It tells the person to guard against the 'end-of-diet mindset'—'now the job is done, and I can return to my old diet'. This phase emphasizes whole, unprocessed foods, but the basic low-carbohydrate character continues.

The Atkins diet and the 'low-carb craze' reached its peak in the US in 2003–2004. Like all lopsided fad diets, the Atkins diet also has had its rise and fall. Its limited success with the overweight is possibly due to the fact that being an unaccustomed and monotonous diet, a person cannot eat too much of it. Second, fats and proteins take longer to digest than carbohydrates. Therefore, a person on this diet does not feel hungry between meals. But the safety of the Atkins diet is controversial. Therefore, it is still prudent to lose weight on a low-calorie, healthy and balanced diet, along with moderate exercise.

Comment on the dictum, 'A healthy diet has a variety of foods'.

In general, variety is desirable because the nutrients missing in one food can be easily obtained from another. However, one should keep two things in mind. First, the variety should be judiciously chosen—any indiscriminate assembly of foods will not ensure adequate nutrition. Second, variety beyond a point may promote overeating ('let me take a bit of everything'), and consequently, weight gain.

On the one hand, milk is said to be a complete food; on the other hand, now, many consider milk to be harmful. Why is there so much controversy about a food that has been consumed for millennia?

The truth possibly lies somewhere between the extremes. Milk alone is suitable as a food only for infants up to about six months of age. Milk is not a complete food for adults, but is acceptable in moderation as part of a diet containing a variety of foods. Some adults find it hard to digest milk because of its lactose content. They can get the benefits of milk from curd, which has much less lactose. Milk is the only source of vitamin B_{12} for vegetarians, and a major source of vitamin D. Milk is considered essential for getting calcium, but the amount of calcium that is really necessary can be obtained from plant foods. Although ragi is rich in calcium, the really necessary amount of calcium can also be obtained from a mixture of other grains, fruits and vegetables that are consumed regularly in predictable amounts far more commonly than ragi. Too much of calcium can even be harmful: it has been linked with osteoporosis and vitamin D deficiency. Regarding the harmful effects of milk, they are controversial, but certainly possible. For example, milk has been linked to Type 1 Diabetes in children, and also to cancer of the prostate. Some of the harmful effects of milk are attributable to the antibiotics, hormones and other drugs that are given to milk-producing cattle. The harmful effects of milk may have been exaggerated by those who are opposed to consumption of milk on ethical grounds. Their arguments do have some validity because milk production is today an industry, and therefore, cattle often receive an unfair deal. This is quite in contrast with the days when the cow was a part of the Indian family, and was respected like the mother. Therefore, the ethical code which we have inherited from that era may not be valid any more. But nutritionally speaking, milk remains an almost essential item of the diet, at least for vegetarians. In view of that, there is a strong case for working towards humane treatment of cattle belonging to the milk industry, and minimizing the use of chemicals for the sake of improving the yield. Besides that, we should also make a conscious effort to consume only as much milk as is essential, which is about one quarter of a litre a day.

Are sprouts better than the corresponding cooked grain?

Yes, sprouts are better for at least two reasons. First, the vitamin content of grains goes up during germination. Second, sprouts are digestible, and therefore, need not be cooked. Cooking brings down the vitamin content of foods.

Is non-vegetarian food essential for good health?

No, it is just as possible to be healthy and strong on a vegetarian diet as on a non-vegetarian one. On the contrary, several much-needed anti-infective, anti-cancer and antioxidant chemicals are found only in plant foods, while some undesirable cancer-inducing substances are found in animal foods.

Are there any nutrients that non-vegetarian foods have but vegetarian foods do not? How can vegetarians get these nutrients?

There are four such nutrients:

1. Cholesterol: Cholesterol is not a dietary requirement because the body can manufacture all the cholesterol that it needs.
2. Vitamin A: The beta-carotene in plant foods (such as carrot, papaya, mango and green leafy vegetables) can substitute for vitamin A.
3. Vitamin D: Exposure to sunshine can substitute for vitamin D. But since exposure to sunshine is often inadequate, vegetarians depend upon milk and milk products for their supply of vitamin D. If that is considered inadequate, a low-dose vitamin D supplement may be taken.
4. Vitamin B_{12}: Vegetarians depend upon milk and milk products for their supply of vitamin B_{12}. If

that is considered inadequate, a supplement may be taken. The supplementation need not be very frequent because the body can store up to three years' requirement of vitamin B_{12}.

Are there any nutrients that vegetarian foods have but non-vegetarian foods do not?

Yes, plenty. The most important among them are carbohydrates, which are present in milk but not in eggs or meat. There are also hundreds of phytochemicals that are found only in plants (See Chapter 7). But this question is somewhat redundant, especially in India, where even non-vegetarians generally eat plenty of plant foods in addition to the non-vegetarian items.

What is the place of eggs in one's daily diet?

Except for the absence of carbohydrates, eggs have almost all the other important nutrients. Therefore, they are a value addition to the diet of a growing child. But their place in the diet of an adult is optional. If a person has a high blood cholesterol level, or a tendency in that direction, eggs should be avoided. If a person has a moral objection to taking eggs, it is reassuring to know that children as well as adults can be healthy without eating eggs.

What is the place of nuts in a balanced diet?

Nuts are high fat foods, and are therefore energy-dense. 1 gram of nuts typically gives about 6 Calories. This is also true of pistachio, the so-called 'skinny nut'. This is a fact of primary importance because it is very easy to overeat in case of nuts and become overweight. Being overweight is itself a major health risk. The type of fats the nuts contain, and all the other beneficial substances that they contain, cannot compensate fully for being overweight. To put it in practical terms, twelve walnut halves, twelve almonds or twenty peanuts weigh 25 grams, and give about 150 Calories, which is the same as the Calories in one banana, or one and a half chapattis. Therefore, nuts have to be compensated for either by removing something else of equivalent calorific value from the diet, or by exercising. A brisk twenty-five-minute walk will burn off 150 Calories; in short, walking for one minute will compensate for 1 gram of nuts. Although nuts are not an essential part of a balanced diet, they are an acceptable food. Among nuts, walnuts and almonds are more 'heart-friendly' than most other nuts, provided we do not eat so many of them as to grow fat.

What is junk food?

Junk food is food that is unhealthy but popular. It is popular because it is palatable, convenient and those who profit from its sale ensure that it is also attractive. Junk foods generally have refined grains, high fat, high sugar and very little of vegetables, if at all, but may have meat, additives and preservatives. These foods overwhelm the appetite, and therefore, leave little room for healthy foods. Further, being palatable, these foods promote overeating and weight gain. Finally, some of the constituents of these foods, such as trans fats, cholesterol or the added chemicals, might affect health adversely.

Is it permissible to mix carbohydrates and proteins in the same meal?

This is not a frequently asked question. But the reason I have included it is that I recently saw a young well-educated man having only dal and curd at lunch, although rice, chapattis and bread were also available. When I asked him why, he said that he was consuming only proteins at lunch, and that he would take only carbohydrates at dinner. When I again asked him why, he said that he had read somewhere on the Internet that that is the healthy way to eat. He was patently wrong on several counts. First, what he was eating was also a mixture of carbohydrates and proteins: dal has 60 per cent carbohydrate, and only 20 per cent protein. What he will eat at dinner is also a mixture of carbohydrates and proteins: cereals like wheat or rice have 70 per cent carbohydrate, and 10 per cent protein. Second, cereal and pulse proteins together give us good quality protein, and having them during the same meal is therefore a healthy practice. Third, our digestive system is smart—it does not get confused by a mixture of nutrients. Finally, everything that is on the Internet is not necessarily correct.

Food combinations, which may be harmful, are very few, and the modern science of nutrition knows hardly any. Ayurveda does have the concept of incompatible foods, or *viruddhahar*, which will be discussed in the next chapter.

How safe is the microwave oven for heating food?

This question has two aspects. The first concerns the effect of heating food in a microwave oven on its nutrient content. Such effects are both favourable and adverse, but neither is probably significant enough to have serious consequences. Food gets heated in the microwave oven to a lower temperature and for a shorter time, which reduces the loss of some heat-labile nutrients such as vitamin C. Less heating also means that food does not get burnt, and since some of the burnt food may be carcinogenic, this is also an advantage. Among the adverse effects is loss of about one-third of the vitamin B_{12} content of the food, due to the active form of the vitamin getting converted into an inactive form during microwaving. Another disadvantage of microwaving is that the heating may not be adequate to sterilize food that is contaminated with harmful germs. This could be an important consideration while reheating stored food.

The second aspect concerns the effect of exposure to microwave radiation on one's health. First, the exposure is minimal because the microwaves remain confined to the oven. Second, the radiation is different in character from X-rays, and is non-carcinogenic. In short, there is at present no well-established effect of using the microwave oven to either encourage or discourage its use.

SUMMARY

1. A diet, which is satisfactory from the scientific point of view, is called a balanced diet. A balanced diet is a vegetarian diet (or at least predominantly so), which contains:

(a) A mixture of cereals and pulses, consumed whole (unrefined) as far as possible, as the staple food.

(b) Five helpings a day of fruits and vegetables, specially green leafy vegetables.

(c) Milk or milk products in moderation.

(d) Spices in moderation.

(e) Moderate quantity of judiciously chosen fats.

(f) Sugar and salt in moderation.

2. For losing weight, the best treatment has two time-honoured components: eating less and exercising more. In general, everything that a person eats should be reduced in quantity, with greater emphasis on sweets and high-fat foods. To ensure that the person does not remain hungry in spite of reducing the energy intake, the quantity of fruits and uncooked vegetables should be increased. Further, the person should cultivate the habits of eating slowly and chewing food well. The sequence in which a person eats various items of the meal can also help. Regarding exercise, it is desirable to both incorporate it in daily life, and to create a special slot for it. Crash diets, yo-yo dieting and fad diets are all less effective in the long run, and may also be unsafe.

9
Old Is Gold

For an optimal dietary regimen one should combine a sattvic diet with a diet appropriate for one's doshic types.

DAVID FRAWLEY

The modern science of nutrition has discovered with great accuracy the chemical nature and metabolic functions of nutrients, the nutrient composition of foods and also how much of each nutrient a person needs. But it still has, essentially, a 'one size fits all' approach. Because of this, every 60 kg, 1.6 metre tall, moderately active man is considered to have almost the same nutritional requirements throughout the year, anywhere in the world. This is quite a contrast with the Ayurvedic approach, which considers it necessary to vary the diet according to the constitution of the individual, the season and the place where the person lives. Further, Ayurveda also gives considerable importance to factors such as the frequency and timing of meals, the sequence in which various items in a meal should be eaten and which foods should or should not be taken together at the same meal. These are factors which the modern science of nutrition is quite ignorant about. Ayurveda classifies foods not in terms of their nutrient composition as modern nutrition does, but in terms of their characteristics or qualities, such as cold or warm, light or heavy; their effect on the constitution, e.g. pitta-aggravating or pitta-pacifying; and their effect on temperament, e.g. sattva-promoting or tamas-promoting. This is terminology that modern science does not understand. Just because modern science does not know or understand something, it does not necessarily mean that that knowledge is wrong or redundant. Some of the Ayurvedic knowledge is folk wisdom in India, handed down from generation to generation. There is a tendency to turn to this knowledge, particularly in diseases where modern medicine proves either inadequate or unhelpful; and interestingly, this approach often works. Ayurvedic knowledge on nutrition is so vast that it is impossible to compress it in one chapter. This chapter will provide only a glimpse of this ancient wisdom. Readers who want to know more may consult an Ayurvedic text for more details; references to a few have been given at the end of the book.

The constitution in terms of doshas

Each individual is, of course, unique, in the sense that no two individuals are exactly alike. But Ayurveda classifies people into seven broad categories based on the theory that the constitution (prakriti) of an individual is determined by the relative proportion of three humors or doshas: kapha, pitta and vata. Thus, there are three types of prakriti in which one of the doshas is dominant: kapha-dominant, pitta-dominant or vata-dominant. Then there are other three types in which a pair of doshas is dominant: kapha-pitta, kapha-vata or vata-pitta. Finally, there is a type in which the three doshas are almost equal—the samadosha prakriti. The fact that a person has a particular prakriti is just the statement of a fact: it is not something to be proud or ashamed about, because no prakriti is good or bad. The prakriti of an individual is determined at conception, even before birth, and does not change throughout life. Prakriti translates into physical, mental and emotional characteristics, susceptibility to certain diseases and characteristic likes and dislikes for foods.

Table 9.1 Some Characteristics Related to Doshas*

Characteristic	Vata	Pitta	Kapha
Body frame	Thin	Medium	Broad
Body weight	Low	Moderate	Heavy
Response to energy imbalance	Gains weight with difficulty	Gains weight easily, and also loses it easily	Gains weight easily but finds it difficult to lose it
Appetite	Variable	High	Low
Thirst	Variable	High	Low
Activity	Restless and creative	Moderately active. Dynamic and short-tempered	Low activity level. Organized and cool
Foods recommended	Sweet, salty and sour. Heavy foods. All spices in moderation	Sweet, bitter and astringent tastes. Neither too heavy nor very light food. Cooling spices such as coriander, turmeric and fennel. Avoid other spices	Pungent, bitter and astringent tastes. Light foods. All spices in moderation

---

*This information is from the point of view of nutrition, and is not enough for you to determine your prakriti.

Varying the diet according to prakriti

The principles behind varying the diet according to prakriti are:

1. Prakriti leads to certain food preferences.
2. The foods preferred by a person are such that they further increase the dosha(s) already dominant in him.
3. Increasing, or aggravating the dominant dosha(s) is undesirable.
4. Hence, the foods recommended are those which reduce or pacify the dominant dosha(s) of the individual.
5. As a general guide, a person should avoid the foods for which he has a natural liking. That may sound cruel, but it is ancient wisdom! For the sake of staying healthy, a person should at least eat less of the foods he likes, and should not neglect the foods he dislikes.

Based on these principles, a few recommended and avoidable prakriti-specific foods have been listed below:

Foods recommended

When vata is dominant (vata-pacifying foods):

Sweet, sour and salty tastes*. Wheat, rice, ghee, curd, milk mixed with ghee and sugar, bananas, tubers, tomatoes,

---

*Ayurveda recognizes six tastes: sweet, salty, sour, pungent, bitter and astringent. All tastes are necessary, and a good diet has the right balance of all the six.

citrus fruits, sweets, spices in moderation, warm foods such as soups.

When pitta is dominant (pitta-pacifying foods):

Sweet, bitter and astringent tastes. Rice, tubers, fenugreek (methi), bitter gourd (karela), steamed/boiled vegetables, milk, sweets, Indian gooseberry (amla), cool and soothing foods such as buttermilk. Only coriander (dhania), turmeric (haldi) and fennel (saunf) among the spices.

When kapha is dominant (kapha-pacifying foods):

Pungent, bitter and astringent tastes. Rice and dal in moderation, methi, karela and honey. All spices in moderation.

Foods to be avoided

When vata is dominant (vata-aggravating foods):

Pungent, bitter and astringent tastes. Cold and frozen foods, cold drinks, yellow gram (arhar) dal, peas, chillies. Besides, fasting also aggravates vata.

When pitta is dominant (pitta-aggravating foods):

Sour, salty and pungent tastes. Hot and spicy foods. Horsegram (kulthi dal), curd, brinjal, green leaves, sesame (til), non-vegetarian food. However, if pitta is dominant, curd may be consumed, mixed with amla.

When kapha is dominant (kapha-aggravating foods):

Sweet, sour and salty tastes. Cold, heavy and oily foods. Black gram (urad dal), kidney beans (rajmah), curd.

However, if kapha is dominant, curd may be taken with honey.

Varying the diet according to season

Although the constitution of an individual in terms of doshas does not change, there is a systematic shift in doshas with changes in season. The shift is expressed in terms of moderate excess (sanchaya, or accumulation) of a dosha, or heavy excess (prakopa, or vitiation) of a dosha. The vitiated dosha needs to be pacified more vigorously than the accumulated dosha, but even the accumulated dosha cannot be neglected. For example, in the rainy season, vata dosha is vitiated, and pitta accumulated. Hence, the first priority is to pacify vata, but pitta should also be pacified. If that is not done, diseases caused by pitta-dominance might appear or get aggravated in the next season, i.e. autumn, in which pitta is vitiated. Thus, in the rainy season, preference should be given to vata- and pitta-pacifying foods, and then one should shift completely to pitta-pacifying foods by autumn. Using the same principles, the diets good for winters and summers are more suitable for countries with cold and hot climates respectively.

To add a little more complexity to the general principles outlined above, Ayurveda recognizes six seasons of about two months each. Further, the last two weeks of a season (ritu) and the first two weeks of the next season are a transitional period, or ritusandhi. The dietary practices should also change gradually during the transitional period. The six seasons and the corresponding dietary recommendations have been outlined in Table 9.2.

Table 9.2 Seasonal Dietary Recommendations

Season	Dominant Dosha	Digestive Fire/ Strength	Dietary Recommendations
Shishira (Late winter) Jan-Feb[1]	Kapha[2]	Strong	Kapha-pacifying diet. Recommendations same as in early winter. Kapha-aggravating foods to be avoided more scrupulously than in early winter
Vasanta (Spring) March-April	Kapha[3]	Moderate	Kapha-pacifying diet. Take wheat, barley and bengal gram. Avoid heavy foods, sweets and sour foods
Grishma (Summer) May-June	Vata[4]	Weak	Vata-pacifying diet. Take cold, sweet and liquid foods. Take rice with ghee, sattu (ground pulse mixture), sherbets, and cold sweetened milk
Varsha (Rains) July-Aug	Vata[5] Pitta[6]	Weak	Vata- and pitta-pacifying diet. Light food. Pay special attention to food and water hygiene. Avoid drinking too much water. Avoid cold drinks
Sharad (Autumn) Sept-Oct	Pitta[7]	Moderate	Pitta-pacifying diet. Avoid having fried and spicy foods, and curd
Hemanta (Early winter) Nov-Dec	Kapha[8]	Strong	Kapha-pacifying diet. Consume sweet, oily, sour and salty foods. Have milk and milk products. Avoid cold and watery drinks

---

[1]Months correspond roughly to seasons as seen in the planes of the northern parts of India.
[2]dosha accumulation, i.e. moderate excess (sanchaya).
[3]dosha vitiated, i.e. heavy excess (prakopa).
[4]dosha accumulation, i.e. moderate excess (sanchaya).
[5]dosha vitiated, i.e. heavy excess (prakopa).
[6]dosha accumulation, i.e. moderate excess (sanchaya).
[7]dosha vitiated, i.e. heavy excess (prakopa).
[8]dosha accumulation, i.e. moderate excess (sanchaya).

The constitution in terms of temperament

While the constitution in terms of the dominant dosha(s) remains constant throughout life, there is an aspect of the constitution, the temperament, which can be modified by personal effort. The modifiable factors that determine the temperament are the modes of nature, or gunas. Like the doshas, there are three basic gunas—sattva, rajas and tamas—and the temperament depends on the dominant guna(s). Sattva is the principle of knowledge, genuine love and harmony. Rajas expresses itself as activity, desires and intense emotions. Tamas is the principle underlying ignorance and inertia. A sattvic person is typically knowledgeable, responsible, considerate and contented. Rajas makes a person hardworking, but greedy and unscrupulous. Tamas makes a person lazy, dull, insincere, slow and inefficient. A person may be predominantly tamasic, rajasic or sattvic, but each one of us has at least a bit of all three. Further, the dominant principle exhibited by a person may not be the same at all times. For example, even a person who is generally lazy may sometimes engage in hectic activity. Finally, what is most important is the fact that the dominant temperament of a person can be changed through knowledge and personal effort. It is desirable to move from tamas towards rajas, and from rajas towards sattva.

The three gunas are often mentioned with reference to food. The Gita says that tamasic persons have a liking for stale and impure food; rajasic persons go for sour, salty and hot (pungent) food; and sattvic persons love healthy, soft and juicy foods (Bhagavad Gita 17:8-10). The verses have subsequently been expanded to name specific foods in each category, and the corresponding foods are popularly called tamasic, rajasic and sattvic foods. It is important to note that in terms of the Gita, it is people who are tamasic, rajasic or sattvic, not the foods. Further, the generalities to which the Gita has confined itself has a significance. A tamasic person is both ignorant and lazy. Because of his ignorance, he does not know which foods are healthy, and therefore, may choose unhealthy foods. Because of his laziness, he is unwilling to put in the effort required for procuring or preparing food. Therefore, he does not seem to mind eating stale food. A rajasic person enjoys strong sensations, and hence chooses foods which provide strong sensory stimulation. A sattvic person knows what is healthy, and loves peace or sweetness in everything. Therefore, he chooses healthy foods, such as soft, sweet and juicy fruits. The psychological element implied in the choice of foods is at least as important as the chemical composition of the food. For example, the sattvic person chooses healthy foods not because of fear of disease or death, but because he likes them better than the alternatives. While he eats fruits and vegetables, his mind does not dwell on omelettes and cutlets. On the other hand, if a tamasic person is provided healthy food, he may eat so much of it out of greed that the net effect may still be unhealthy.

While it is true that temperament, in terms of gunas, determines food preferences, Ayurveda believes that the relationship works both ways: foods can also affect the temperament. Hence, efforts to modify one's temperament should also include attention to the diet. For example, non-violence is a sattvic attribute. Therefore, a sattvic person is likely to prefer vegetarian food. But conversely, turning vegetarian can also promote the growth of sattva in a person.

Sattva-promoting foods

Sattva-promoting foods are recommended for all. The first and foremost feature of a sattvic diet is that it is vegetarian. It includes plenty of fruits and vegetables, preferably organic, and avoids canned and processed foods. The food is pleasant in taste, but not over-sweet; in fact, a balance of all the six tastes is what makes the diet sattvic. Sattvic spices are the mild ones such as ginger (adrak), cinnamon (dalchini) and cardamom (elaichi). Further, sattvic food is freshly cooked, which is not always practical these days. However, one should avoid storing food in the refrigerator for too long.

Rajas-promoting foods

Although sattva is the most desirable mode of nature, rajas also has a place in life, especially for rulers, leaders, administrators and all those who have to think fast, take quick decisions and benefit from being ambitious and goal-oriented. Rajasic foods have a salty, sour or pungent taste, contain an excess of irritant spices like chillies and are hot in temperature.

Tamas-promoting foods

Tamas is an undesirable temperament, and therefore, tamasic foods should be avoided. Irrespective of the food one eats, overeating promotes tamas. Stored, canned, processed, stale, fried and heavy foods also promote tamas. Meat is tamasic and so are refined grains and white sugar.

When, how and how much

Besides what to eat, minor details about factors such as the timing, frequency and sequence are also considered important in Ayurveda. The feeling of fullness is a good guide to the right quantity of food in a meal*. The dictum, as mentioned earlier, is to imagine that the stomach has four compartments. Only two of these should be filled with food, one with water and one should remain empty. In other words, one should end a meal at a point when one still has the capacity to eat some more. The distribution of food among different meals should be guided by the capacity of the digestive system, or the agni (digestive fire). The digestive fire is at its peak between 10 a.m. and 2 p.m. Therefore, the heaviest meal of the day should be during this interval. The total number of meals should be two to three, unless recommended otherwise

---

*Physiologically, this is valid only if the meal has unrefined grains, includes enough of fruits and vegetables and is eaten slowly.

by a doctor. A meal should be consumed only after the previous meal has been digested, and after appetite has returned. This happens if the interval between meals is at least three hours, preferably more than four. Therefore, munching on snacks between meals should be avoided as much as possible, preferably entirely. If one feels hungry between meals, a fruit is the best option. A certain amount of regularity in terms of timings of meals and the quantity at each meal is also desirable.

The meal should start with a sweet, with fruit or salad, or with half a glass of water*. The main course of the meal should have salty and sour tastes. Pungent, bitter and astringent tastes should come towards the end. Thus, the meal may end with cardamom (elaichi), cloves (laung), fennel (saunf) or papad. Ideally, every meal should have all the six tastes. Cooking and processing may alter the quality of a food. For example, unripe mango is 'hot' but ripe mango is not, and when mango is converted into 'panna', it becomes 'cold'. Spices, in general, should always be cooked. Either the spices should be heated with a little oil or ghee and then poured over cooked food; or spices should be allowed to simmer as the food is getting cooked.

---

*Physiologically, all three make sense. A sweet raises the blood sugar promptly, and will, therefore, prevent overeating. Fruit and salad take time to eat, and are also filling. Therefore, these items at the beginning of the meal also avoid overeating. Water is also filling, and therefore prevents overeating.

Food interactions

It is good to have a variety of foods at every meal, but some combinations are considered incompatible. Mixing foods that do not go well together is called viruddhahar (literally, contrary diet). Some such combinations are well-known. For example, most people in India avoid consuming fish and milk during the same meal. But even the cereal and milk combination, which is a popular breakfast, is considered viruddhahar in Ayurveda. In fact, milk is considered incompatible with cereals, dals, uncooked food (e.g. salad, fruit, sprouts), sour and salty foods and all non-vegetarian foods. This essentially rules out drinking milk with any meal; thus, the only time left for having milk is as a bedtime drink (a few hours after an early dinner), or as the sole item at breakfast. A few other examples of viruddhahar are:

1. Cooked and uncooked foods: Thus the salad or fruit should be finished before the meal; it should not be taken a bit at a time throughout the meal.

2. Hot and cold (in terms of temperature) foods: Thus, a cold drink, ice-cold water, or ice cream are incompatible with a meal; also, tea and a cold drink in quick succession are incompatible with each other.

3. Black gram (urad dal) and radish (mooli).

4. Ghee and honey in equal quantity: both ghee and honey are commonly considered health foods. There have been cases of people taking a spoon of ghee and a spoon of honey one after another

to get their quota of health food for the day and landing in trouble.

The effects of taking incompatible foods include skin diseases (e.g. rashes and leucoderma), piles and severe allergic reactions, occasionally even leading to death.

Closing thoughts

The reader now has far too many guidelines on what to eat. The diet should be based on prakriti; the diet should be sattvic; the diet should be appropriate to the season; the meal should include all six tastes but it should not include incompatible foods; and last but not least, the diet should take into account the gender, physical activity level, dietary habits, occupation and health status of the individual. On top of all this, it is difficult to ignore the recommendations based on the modern science of nutrition and the results of continuing research. If I have created the confusion, it is my responsibility to at least try to clear it up.

The main point is that there is no essential contradiction between all these guidelines. To start with, one may use the modern science of nutrition to frame a balanced diet as outlined towards the end of Chapter 8. Then, using each of the guidelines in this chapter, one may emphasize a few foods and restrict a few others. Thus, giving a thought to doshas, gunas and the six tastes can help us give a certain tilt to the basic balanced diet. Further, the direction of the tilt may be different for different members of the family, because their prakritis are unlikely to be exactly the same. For example, starting with the same basic diet for the whole family, those with vata dominance may take additional ghee; those with pitta dominance may take an extra glass of buttermilk (chhachh) and some fennel (saunf), coriander (dhania) or amla; and those with kapha dominance may add some black pepper (kali mirch) or dry ginger (saunth/adrak) powder to their food. If a particular food is appropriate for the prakriti of the individual but is not sattva-promoting, that food can be restricted in favour of a dosha-appropriate sattvic food. In winters, one may drink hot soup or herbal tea, and in summers a sherbet or mango panna. In order to respect the concept of incompatible foods, one may have water or tea instead of milk along with the parantha, idli or bread at breakfast. The milk may be shifted to the night, a couple of hours after an early dinner. The vata-dominant person may have the bedtime milk hot, while the pitta-dominant person should cool it down. In short, the finer points that Ayurveda gives us should be used for fine-tuning the basic balanced diet worked out earlier on the basis of the modern science of nutrition.

It is often suggested that Ayurvedic concepts should be examined by the methods of modern science. Behind this suggestion is the fond hope, in fact usually a firm belief, that the examination will revalidate these concepts, thereby lending them greater acceptance and respectability. While the suggestion is inspired by the patriotic feelings of Indians as well as the urge for contributing to human welfare, it is not easy to implement. The positive effect of adhering to the multiple guidelines of Ayurveda, or the negative effect of violating them, is likely to be small and subtle and may take several years to manifest. Scientific studies cannot easily detect such small and subtle long-term effects. Also, the number of factors that could affect the outcome, and the number of outcome variables in such studies, would be extremely large. Going by the analytical approach of modern science, looking at one factor at a time would not only be inappropriate but also very time-consuming: it could easily keep hundreds of teams of scientists busy for centuries. Add to that the classification of subjects into at least seven subgroups based on their prakriti, and we have an enormous task and extremely complicated data in store, if ever such studies are undertaken.

The next question that may be asked is how Ayurveda acquired all this knowledge if it is so difficult to arrive at. The rational answer to this question is that it has been arrived at by trial and error as a result of natural experiments that have been going on in large populations for millennia. The non-rational, or rather supra-rational (to use an expression of Sri Aurobindo's) explanation is that the pioneers of Ayurveda were not ordinary physicians or scientists but rishis (sages). Ayurveda is, in fact, an Upaveda (subsidiary Veda) of the *Atharvaveda,* one of the four Vedas. Rishis have access to knowledge from planes higher than the mental. Hence, Ayurveda is also revealed knowledge, knowledge revealed to the ancient Indian spiritual masters. Although not rational,

I find this explanation more plausible than the trial-and-error theory. The remarkable fact is that so much of the knowledge has survived the passage of thousands of years, and it works. If a person taking a dosha-inappropriate diet has a disease to which persons with his prakriti are more susceptible, giving him a diet which pacifies his dominant dosha does help in arresting the ferocity of the disease.

Frequently Asked Questions

What is the difference between an Ayurvedic diet and a yogic diet?

There is considerable overlap between the two, but there is also a difference. Ayurveda is a system of medicine. Therefore, the primary aim of an Ayurvedic diet is promotion, preservation and restoration of health, including spiritual health. Thus, in Ayurveda, spiritual growth is an aspect of total health and well-being. On the other hand, yoga is a physical and mental discipline designed for spiritual growth. Therefore, although a yogic diet also aims at good health, its primary concern is the effect it might have on spiritual growth. Hence, in yogic diets, the promotion of sattva is the dominant consideration. Ayurveda also favours sattvic foods, not so much for their spiritual effects, but primarily because sattvic foods pacify all doshas. The primary consideration in Ayurvedic diets is to reduce or pacify the dominant dosha. Ayurveda does not lay stress on reducing attachment to food the way yoga does. In short, the Ayurvedic diet aims at physical health so that the body and mind *can* work in light of the soul. In contrast, yoga aims at a diet that facilitates the process whereby the body and mind *actually* work in light of the soul.

What is the difference between an Ayurvedic diet and a naturopathic diet?

Ayurveda and naturopathy are both systems of medicine, but their underlying philosophies are different. Ayurveda looks upon health as a state of balance of the three doshas; imbalance leads to disease. Naturopathy does not have a clear, unanimously agreed upon underlying doctrine, but disease being due to toxins or 'morbid matter' is a recurring theme. A wide variety of practitioners, each practising different modes of treatment, call themselves naturopaths. What unites all naturopaths is their strong aversion to allopathic drugs and surgery. For many naturopaths, diet is the major form of therapy. They classify therapeutic diets into (a) eliminative diets, which are liquid diets that are assumed to remove some hypothetical toxins from the body by purging, vomiting, etc.; (b) soothing diets, which have only raw fruits and vegetables; and (c) constructive diets, which have unrefined grains, sprouts and curd. Because of the difference in underlying theories, not only is the approach to diet in Ayurveda and naturopathy quite different, but practitioners of the two systems may sometimes give the exact opposite advice about the same food. On the whole, Ayurvedic diets are more user-friendly. Naturopathic diets tend to be rather monotonous and unpalatable.

What is satmyam?

In Ayurveda, satmyam means 'appropriateness'. 'Satmya diet' is a diet appropriate in terms of prakriti, processing, combination, quantity, place, time, eater and the 'rules of eating' (bhojana-niyama).

What are 'hot' and 'cold' foods?

In Ayurveda, 'hot' or 'cold' refers not to the temperature, but the metabolic effects of a food. There is no known consistent correlate of this concept in modern science, but that does not mean that the concept is wrong.

What is the opinion of Ayurveda about curd?

Curd is an acceptable food, but with a few reservations. First, those having pitta or kapha dominance should avoid it, although they may have chhachh (buttermilk). For similar reasons, curd should not be taken during certain periods of the day, certain seasons or in diseases when pitta or kapha are dominant. Thus, the best time to consume curd is between 2 p.m. and 6 p.m. Second, curd should not be taken if it is 'under-formed' (hypo-mature) or 'sour' (hyper-mature). Third, curd should not be taken at night.

Comment on the proverb, 'Breakfast like a king, lunch like a prince, dine like a pauper'.

This proverb is often misinterpreted. It does not mean that breakfast should be the heaviest meal. Which king would eat more than his son? He would give the richest foods to the son, and the young growing boy, with his enormous appetite, would eat more than the father. Interpreted in this way, the proverb agrees with the Ayurvedic principles that the heaviest meal of the day should be lunch.

What does Ayurveda have to say about the proverb, 'After lunch, rest a while; after supper, walk a while'.

The proverb is essentially right because in hot climates, as in India, it is much better to have some rest after lunch than to go out for a walk in the sun. However, Ayurveda does have some elaborate guidelines on the post-lunch period. Immediately after a meal, especially after lunch, which is the heaviest meal, one should sit erect, preferably in vajrasana (thunderbolt posture or the namaaz pose) for about ten minutes (less, if it becomes painful). Then one should walk slowly for about ten minutes. After that, one should lie down on the left side, for about ten minutes. Sleeping during the daytime is appropriate only in summers. The old and infirm, however, may sleep during the daytime throughout the year.

SUMMARY

1. Ayurveda considers it necessary to vary the diet according to the constitution of the individual, the season and the place where the person lives. Further, Ayurveda also attributes considerable importance to factors such as the frequency and timing of meals, the sequence in which various items in a meal should be eaten and which foods

should or should not be taken together at the same meal. These are factors which the modern science of nutrition is quite ignorant about.

2. Ayurveda classifies people in terms of their constitution (prakriti), which is determined by the relative proportion of three humors, or doshas: kapha, pitta and vata.

3. The foods preferred by a person further increase, or aggravate, his dominant dosha, which is undesirable. Hence, the foods recommended to a person are those which decrease, or pacify, his dominant dosha. In other words, a person has to learn to like foods, the liking for which does not come naturally to him.

4. Irrespective of prakriti, sattvic foods are preferable to rajasic and tamasic foods.

5. Sattvic foods, apart from their positive spiritual effects, pacify all doshas.

6. Besides selecting the dominant, dosha-pacifying sattvic foods, one should pay attention to season and the compatibility of foods taken at the same meal.

7. Besides what one eats, also important are factors such as which meal it is, the sequence in which various items are consumed, the quantity of each item and the total quantity of food consumed and the attitude towards food.

10
From Knowledge to Wisdom

Knowledge comes, but wisdom lingers.

ALFRED TENNYSON

How food affects us depends on what we eat, how much we eat and the attitude with which we eat. The focus of the previous chapters has been on 'what' and 'how much'. In this chapter, we shall turn to the significance of the attitude towards food. Two contrasting attitudes to food are summed up in the popular expression, 'Living to eat, or eating to live'. The 'living to eat' attitude makes eating the very purpose of life. This is the attitude of a person who lives a superficial life. To him, the pleasure of eating is a major justification and compensation for the effort involved in making a living. He does not see much meaning in life beyond feeding, breeding and sleeping. To him, it does not matter that this is the way animals also live. Whether human life has a unique purpose is a question that he does not take seriously; in fact, the question may not occur to him at all. In contrast, the 'eating to live' attitude considers food to be merely a necessity for staying alive. This is the attitude of a person whose life has some depth. To him, the purpose of life may range from the joy of getting to the joy of giving, but one thing he knows is that joy does not reside in the food that he eats. He may seek joy in work, wealth, name and fame, power and position, or in social service. But the highest wisdom passed down the ages by spiritual masters is that none of these is adequate for finding fulfillment in life, because all of them address the needs of only the body, mind and intellect. Fulfillment comes when the body, mind and intellect are used merely as instruments to meet the spiritual need for growth of consciousness. Returning to the point of this chapter, when we decide that the purpose of life is not limited to enjoying food, we can graduate to the attitude of eating to live, which is the attitude that will occupy us for the rest of this chapter.

What about taste?

Food that is good to taste appeals to the senses, no matter what the attitude to food is. To get some pleasure from food that tastes good, even if it is only a fleeting pleasure, is also a physiological fact. If one treats food as a necessity, not as a pleasure, how does one handle the inevitable pleasure that comes from tasty food? First, by training one's mind to not long for food that tastes good. We should have better and higher goals than good food to think about. Second, when we have the choice between something that tastes good but is unhealthy and something that does not taste so good but is healthy, we should go for the latter. Finally, when we eat something that tastes good, we should not eat too much of it out of greed.

Let us now reflect on how we develop ideas about what tastes good. These ideas are not inborn; they are shaped by our environment. If a child is being fussy about eating, his parents try to entice him by offering something that *they* think tastes good. Thus, in Bengal, they might offer him a rasgulla; in Gujarat, shrikhand; and in Delhi, ice cream. As these children grow up, they get conditioned to think of these different foods when they are asked which food they like the most. This conditioning, initiated in childhood, is sustained throughout life by at least three routes. One, as adults, these persons now do to their children what their parents did to them, and in the process also strengthen their own conditioning. Two, their parents treat them like children throughout life. Even if a fifty-year-old visits her mother, the mother tries to feed 'her child' the same things that she taught her to like as a five-year-old. Three, the conditioning can be so strong that even if a person has taught himself to look beyond taste, he behaves as if it is his duty to find a particular food very tasty! Thus, there is nothing absolute about what tastes good. We first learn to like certain foods, and then continue liking them without giving it a thought.

The other side of the coin is that conditioning can be turned around to become an aid to healthy eating. Carrot is sweet; and so are apples, grapes and pears. There is no absolute reason why this sweetness is less pleasant than that of ice cream. If a person makes a conscious effort to appreciate the sweetness of fruits, he can get conditioned to find fruits very tasty. When some people give up sugar for health reasons, initially, they find their tea tasteless. They keep reminding themselves that the sugarless tea is tasteless but is better for their health. Finally, they reach a point when they find that tea both tasty and healthy. Now, if somebody serves them tea with sugar, they do not like its taste. Thus, it is possible to decondition oneself by conscious effort. It is also possible to recondition oneself so that what is good (shreyas) also becomes pleasant (preyas). When Mahatma Gandhi went to England, he initially found it very difficult to put up with the monotonous and insipid vegetables that were all that he could manage by way of vegetarian food. But his commitment to vegetarianism and self-control raised him to a level where he started liking even boiled spinach. While narrating these incidents in his autobiography, he wrote, 'Many such experiments taught me that the real seat of taste is not the tongue but the mind'*.

Suppression or mastery?

All wisdom traditions agree on the need to rise above flimsy, fragile and futile sensory pleasures, and instead

---

*Gandhi, M.K. *An Autobiography or The Story of My Experiments with Truth*. New Delhi: Rupa Publications, 2011.

concentrate on steady and meaningful goals. However, they do not agree on the way this may be done; there are at least two ways to do it. One of the ways is to kill the desire for sensory pleasures by keeping away from them, using brute will power (nigraha). The other way is to gain mastery by overcoming attachment to the object of desire (samyama). Let us examine both these methods as applied to food, since eating is one of the most difficult among the sensory pleasures to overcome.

It is certainly possible to use strong determination to keep completely away from all food that tastes good. Using strong willpower, it is even possible to sustain the abstinence for very long periods. But if, behind the heroic effort, there is only the desire to demonstrate one's willpower, what sustains the abstinence is the admiration it invites and the egoistic satisfaction it provides. The desire does not really disappear; it is merely pushed aside*. The person keeps reminding himself, 'I cannot overcome the desire, but my willpower is so strong that

---

*If the desire stays but is not satisfied, that can also lead to mental stress. The person may be eating fruits and vegetables, but his mind may be dwelling on omelettes and cutlets. The person may be fasting, but his mind may be dwelling on what he will eat when he breaks the fast. These are stressful mental states. Mental stress is a major contributor to lifestyle diseases. Therefore, if the attachment to food has not been overcome, the stress due to missing the wrong foods may do more harm than the good resulting from eating the right foods. That is why this chapter is not merely philosophy; it has practical implications.

I will not yield to it.' The result is that this person keeps away from tasty food, but is thinking about it all the time. He thrives on a perverse satisfaction derived from classifying all the foods presented to him in terms of taste, and leaving out those that taste good. In other words, the person still pays attention to taste, perhaps more than average attention, but makes an unusual choice by choosing the unpleasant-tasting foods. Thus, he has failed to overcome his attachment to food; he has merely replaced a positive attachment with a negative attachment. But negative attachment is still an attachment, and therefore, bondage. In short, mere suppression does not fulfill the objective of overcoming attachment to food so that the mind can be free to seek higher goals. So long as attachment continues, whether positive or negative, the mind cannot focus on higher goals.

The other method aimed at mastering the desire for food is based on overcoming the attachment to food rather than physically keeping away from it. This attitude follows inner development in two directions. First, the person realizes the true purpose of food, which is to nourish the body rather than to please the palate. Second, the person has a higher goal to aspire for. The result is that the person develops a tendency to think less and less about food, including its taste. If he gets food that tastes good, he enjoys it. But he is not attached to the taste, he does not make special efforts to seek it, he does not long for it. If he does not get food that tastes good, he does not miss it. In short, his happiness does not depend on the taste of the food. Not being at the mercy of a sensory pleasure for happiness is true liberation. Thus, acquiring mastery over a sensory pleasure is an inside-out approach. It consists of an inner change, which is reflected in an outer change. The inner change is lack of attachment. The outer change is not caring for the taste of food. As Sri Aurobindo said, 'If I get, I take; if I don't get, I shall not mind'. If a person is offered a lavish, palatable meal, and he makes a fuss, saying, 'I do not eat sweets. I do not eat spices. I do not eat fried foods. I love only fruits and vegetables', it is generally more an expression of the sattvic ego than mastery over taste. Yes, sattva also has an ego, and that is why the ideal of the Gita is to go beyond the three gunas. As long as the attachment stays, physically keeping away from sensory pleasures does not serve any spiritual purpose. Once the attachment goes, keeping away from the pleasures is not necessary but the tendency to keep away from them comes automatically. There is an expression in the *Isha Upanishad*, '*tena tyaktena bhunjithaa*', which means 'renounce and enjoy'. It may be asked how one can enjoy if one has renounced. Here, renunciation refers to inner renunciation, or giving up of attachment. In this sense, one can truly enjoy only if one has renounced! With inner renunciation, the sensory pleasure, which has come without seeking or struggle, can be enjoyed without worrying about how long it will last. One can simply enjoy it while it lasts, and then forget about it.

Mealtime yoga

One of the celebrated quotes of Sri Aurobindo is 'All life is yoga', which means that all life is an opportunity for the practise of yoga. How can mealtime also be such an opportunity? One way is to start meals with a prayer—silent or loud—not as a ritual, but as a sincere expression of gratitude and reaffirmation. In a world still inhabited by millions who are not sure of the next meal, getting food is a privilege for which we should be grateful to the Divine. Not only getting food, but even having an appetite, the capacity to eat and the ability to digest are privileges. There are patients who have food available but are unable to eat or swallow it, and therefore, have to be fed by means of a tube going through the nose down to the stomach. Mealtimes are also opportunities to remind ourselves that food is not a sensory pleasure, but a requirement for survival and physical fitness.

This reminder helps us choose the right foods in just the right quantity, neither too much nor too little. Mealtimes may also be used for reaffirming that the purpose of staying physically fit is to maintain a body that can serve as an efficient instrument of the Divine. Hence, at mealtimes, one may pray that the meal be translated into a healthy body, so that one can make best use of the privilege of serving as a channel of the divine force in the material world. The prayer at mealtimes can extend beyond oneself to include the company one has during the meal. One may thank the Divine for the company of near and dear ones, and pray for their health and well-being. There is no bar on including even items unrelated to food in the mealtime prayer.

After the prayer comes eating. As with other activities, eating should be a conscious activity—slow, deliberate, peaceful and fully aware. This will enhance the joy of eating, avoid overeating as well as accidents (such as food entering the wrong passage) and improve digestion. Therefore, one should restrict talking to a minimum while eating, eat sitting down rather than standing and certainly not eat while walking.

The meal should also end with a prayer—it may be a short one. The shortest and best prayer has just two words: thank you. Spoken from the heart, it encompasses all other prayers.

Closing thoughts

Food can be looked at in many ways. On an ascending scale, food is a sensory pleasure, a source of nutrients necessary for life, a product of the hard work put in by a farmer, an expression of Nature's love, a part of the mahayajna (grand give and take, or recycling) that the world is and a manifestation of the Divine. All matter is a manifestation of the Divine, but since our food keeps us alive, it is easier to see the Divine in food than in other materials. The life force that makes us seek food, eat it, digest it and utilize it is also a manifestation of the Divine. The life force packed in the food, which in turn generates the life force by which we stay alive and work, is also a manifestation of the Divine. A thinking, self-healing machine comparable to man, which runs efficiently on a simple renewable fuel like foodgrains, is yet to be invented by man. It is only appropriate that man surrenders his will to the divine will, uses his body–mind complex for what the Divine expects of him and consecrate all his work by offering it to the Divine. As the Gita says: 'Brahman (the Divine) is the giving. Brahman is the food offering. By Brahman it is offered to the Brahman-fire (the digestive system). To Brahman goes he who perceives only Brahman in his actions' (4:24).

SUMMARY

1. How food affects us depends on what we eat, how much we eat and the attitude with which we eat.
2. Time-honoured wisdom traditions tell us that the right attitude to food is: eat to live.
3. Mastering the desire for food should be based on overcoming the attachment to food rather than killing the desire. The inner change should then get reflected in outer change.
4. The mealtime prayer is a good opportunity to remind ourselves about the right attitude to food.

Acknowledgements

I am grateful to:

- Dr Surinder Katoch, MD (Ayurveda), for going through Chapter 9, and making many valuable changes and additions,
- D. K. Singhal, for typing several chapters accurately, promptly and happily,
- Kapish Mehra of Rupa Publications, for approaching me to contribute to their series on health,
- The participants in my courses, camps and lectures for making me aware of the common questions and misconceptions and
- Last but not least, to the Divine for that unseen Hand, which initiates, sustains and supports all human endeavour.

Further Reading

Dahanukar, Sharadini and Urmila Thatte. *Ayurveda Unravelled.* New Delhi: National Book Trust, India, 1996.

Frawley, David. *Ayurveda and the Mind: The healing of consciousness.* Delhi: Motilal Banarsidass, 1998.

———. *Yoga and Ayurveda: Self-healing and self-realization.* Delhi: Motilal Banarsidass, 2000.

Sharma, Priya Vrat. *Essentials of Ayurveda: Text and translation of Sodasangahrdayam.* Delhi: Motilal Banarsidass, 2nd edition, 1998.

The classical texts of Ayurveda, *Charaka Samhita*, *Susruta Samhita* and *Ashtanga Sangraha* are in Sanksrit, but their translations into English and several Indian languages are available.

The website *http://ayurveda-foryou.com* also has plenty of useful information on Ayurveda.

www.ingramcontent.com/pod-product-compliance
Lightning Source LLC
Chambersburg PA
CBHW031516270326
41930CB00006B/423